Nursing Informatics

For Churchill Livingstone

Publisher: Mary C. Law
Project Editor: Dinah Thom
Senior Project Controller: Neil A. Dickson
Project Controller: Nicky S. Haig
Sales Promotion Executive: Hilary Brown

Nursing Informatics

Edited by

Paul Wainwright SRN DipN DANS MSc RNT
Programme Manager: Graduate Studies,
Mid and West Wales College of Nursing and Midwifery,
University College of Swansea, Swansea, UK

CHURCHILL LIVINGSTONE
EDINBURGH LONDON MADRID MELBOURNE NEW YORK AND TOKYO 1994

CHURCHILL LIVINGSTONE
Medical Division of Longman Group UK Limited

Distributed in the United States of America by Churchill Livingstone Inc., 650 Avenue of the Americas, New York, N.Y. 10011, and by associated companies, branches and representatives throughout the world.

© Longman Group UK Limited 1994

All rights reserved. No part of this publication may be reproduced, stored in a retrieval system, or transmitted in any form or by any means, electronic, mechanical, photocopying, recording or otherwise, without either the prior permission of the publishers (Churchill Livingstone, Robert Stevenson House, 1-3 Baxter's Place, Leith Walk, Edinburgh EH1 3AF), or a licence permitting restricted copying in the United Kingdom issued by the Copyright Licensing Agency Ltd, 90 Tottenham Court Road, London, W1P 9HE.

First published 1994

ISBN 0 443 04705 7

British Library of Cataloguing in Publication Data
A catalogue record for this book is available from the British Library.

Library of Congress Cataloging in Publication Data
Nursing informatics / edited by Paul Wainwright.
    p.   cm.
Includes index.
1. Nursing informatics. I. Wainwright, Paul.
[DNLM: 1. Medical Informatics–nurses' instruction.   2. Nursing. WY 26.5 N9738 1994]
RT50.5.N866 1994
610.73'0285–dc20
DNLM/DLC
for Library of Congress   93-36803

The publisher's policy is to use paper manufactured from sustainable forests

Produced by Longman Singapore Publishers (Pte) Ltd
Printed in Singapore

Contents

Contributors vii

Preface ix

1. Towards a founding principle of nursing informatics   1
   Jos Aarts

2. From village to big city: nursing informatics   17
   Pieter Verduin, Paul Epping

3. Formalising nursing knowledge   29
   Maureen Theobald

4. Formalising nursing knowledge: translating nurses describing and thinking about their patients   41
   Alan Hyslop

5. The need for information requirements analysis and evaluation   71
   Wendy King

6. Information requirement analysis and evaluation   87
   Nicola Eaton

7. Nursing information in support of clinical practice   101
   Derek Hoy

8. PAWMEX—an expert system prototype to assist pressure sore risk assessment and wound management   115
   Norman Woolley

9. Computers' use for professional practice: what do nurses need to know?   129
   Susan Grobe

10. Information technology and the curriculum 139
    Mary Chambers

11. The student nurse's use of information technology
    —a Welsh perspective 159
    Pauline Tang

12. Ethical implications of nursing informatics 177
    Paul Wainwright

Index 193

Contributors

Jos E. C. M. Aarts MSc
Consultant/researcher, CAUSA, Centre for Informatics in Health and Welfare, Hogeschool Eindhoven, Eindhoven, The Netherlands

Mary Chambers BEd(Hons) RGN RMN RNT
Senior Lecturer, Department of Nursing, University of Ulster, Coleraine, Northern Ireland

Nicola M. Eaton BSc(Econ)(Hons) RGN RSCN
Lecturer in Nursing, University College of Swansea, Swansea, UK

Paul J. M. M. Epping BC RN
Lecturer in Nursing Informatics and Information Management, Leidse Hogeschool, Leiden, The Netherlands

Susan J. Grobe PhD FAAN
Professor of Nursing; Director, Center for Health Care Research and Evaluation, University of Texas at Austin, School of Nursing, Texas, USA

Derek Hoy RGN RNT BSc(SocSc) MSc(NEd)
Nursing Systems Development, Directorate of Information Services; Management Executive, National Health Service in Scotland, UK

Alan Hyslop RGN RMN MA PhD
Nursing Systems Manager, Directorate of Information Services, National Health Service in Scotland, UK

Wendy King BA MBA RGN RM RHV MIMgt
Senior Consultant, C International Ltd, London, UK

Pauline Chai Tin Tang MN RN RM ONC RCNT CertEd RNT
Nurse Teacher, South East Wales Institute of Nursing and Midwifery Education, University of Wales College of Medicine, University Hospital of Wales, Cardiff, UK

Maureen Theobald MA RGN RCNT RNT DipEd
Principal, Nightingale and Guy's College; Dean of Nursing, UMDS; Chairman, ENB; Non-executive Director, Bromley Health Authority; Honorary Fellow of Faculty, University of Brighton, UK

Pieter J. M. Verduin PT MA PhD
Lecturer in Philosophy of Public Health, Leidse Hogeschool (Leiden Polytechnic), Leiden, The Netherlands

Paul Wainwright SRN DipN DANS MSc RNT
Programme Manager: Graduate Studies, Mid and West Wales College of Nursing and Midwifery, University College of Swansea, Swansea, UK

Norman Woolley RGN DipN MN PGCE RNT
Senior Lecturer in Nursing Studies, Mid Glamorgan College of Nursing and Midwifery, Mid Glamorgan, UK

Preface

Interest in nursing informatics has grown in a remarkable way in the UK in the last few years. However, there remains a lack of literature on the subject, and it is hoped that this book goes some way towards improving that situation.

This book is a product of the European Summer School in Nursing Informatics. The first summer school was held in Leusden, The Netherlands, in 1991, and the second in Stirling, Scotland, in 1992. All of the contributors to the book were involved in the summer school in some way, as tutors, as members of the organising committee, or as delegates. The book is thus also a tribute to the work of these people.

The summer school has been supported from the start by grants from the Erasmus Fund of the European Community, and its success and the production of this book are due in no small measure to the support we have received from a variety of organisations. These include: TDS Healthcare Systems, Atwork, the Digital Equipment Corporation, the Department of Health of the Dutch Government, the English Department of Health, the Scottish Home and Health Department, the National Health Service Training Directorate, the Welsh National Board for Nursing, Midwifery and Health Visiting, the National Board for Nursing, Midwifery and Health Visiting of Northern Ireland, the Leidse Hogeschool, the University of Glasgow, the University of Wales College of Medicine, the University College of Swansea, the University of Ulster at Coleraine, University College Dublin, the University of Brighton, the University of the South Bank, and many others.

1993   P.W.

1

Towards a founding principle of nursing informatics

J. Aarts

Introduction
Medical informatics
Nursing informatics

INTRODUCTION

A reasonable amount of literature about nursing informatics has been published over the past decade. However, most of it deals with practical applications, implicitly assuming some kind of definition of nursing informatics. A review of the literature shows that very few papers deal explicitly with a definition (Graves & Corcoran 1989).

This is, however, not surprising since nursing informatics and medical informatics are young specialities that yet have to develop their own scientific methods.

Chapter 1 will attempt to present a founding principle of nursing informatics by looking at similar approaches in medical informatics and extrapolating from them to the field of nursing. This approach will not be definitive, but I hope that it will stimulate discussion about the true nature of nursing informatics. A clearer vision of nursing informatics will not only provide a direction for research and the development of applications in nursing, but will also set guidelines for education in nursing informatics.

The term 'informatics' originates from French (informatique) and German (Informatik). Collen (1986) even suggests that it originated in the Russian language. The term has been coined to stress the importance of the representation of data and the formalisation of information processing through programming rather than the architecture ('nuts and bolts') of a computer. It is interesting to note that in English-speaking countries it is only in the health care field that the term 'informatics' has become familiar, and that in other areas 'computer science' is being used instead.

Table 1.1   Scope of medical informatics (after Blum 1991)

	1950s	1960s	1970s	1980s
Data applications	Research	Prototype	Mature	Refined
Information applications	Concepts	Research	Prototype	Mature
Knowledge applications	Concepts	Concepts	Research	Prototype

MEDICAL INFORMATICS

Medical informatics emerged as a field in the 1960s. Reichertz is said to have introduced the term in 1969 when he established the Abteilung für Medizinische Informatik (Department of Medical Informatics) at the Hannover Medical School (Möhr 1989).

Blum describes three phases in the development of medical informatics (Blum 1986). The first phase focused on the successful development of data-oriented applications, the second phase on the operational demonstration of information-oriented applications, and the third phase as the conceptual demonstration of knowledge-oriented applications (Table 1.1).

His observation is confirmed by the fact that a number of researchers involved in the origins of medical informatics have their background in the signal-processing community. It must be noted that this description of developments in medical informatics reflects advances in research and, to a lesser extent, the situation in practice. For example, many hospital information systems are still based on the original needs for computing in hospitals which were primarily concerned with financial accounting. Systems that support health care practice are still not abundant.

To begin with medical informatics was very automation-oriented, and gradually it became customary to view the computer in medicine not as an object of research but rather as a tool of health practice. From that viewpoint one started to look at medicine as an object of research to study problems, the choice of which was closely related to the fact that the use of computers always requires a formalised approach.

With the help of Table 1.1 the history of medical informatics can be described. In the data applications phase much work was done in the field of signal and image processing. For example, computer methods were being developed to analyse ECGs and EEGs, and these developments gained impetus when small dedicated computers became available. The results of this research now lie at the heart of the modern monitoring systems used in intensive care departments. A similar development can be seen with respect to image processing where smears and tissue samples are now routinely analysed by computers linked to optical scanners.

The hospital information system that supports health care is the result of the information applications phase. Weed (1969) published a seminal book in which he described the necessity for a problem-oriented approach to health care delivery, arguing for the use of a structured database to record the problems, assessment, interventions and outcomes because of the complexity of medical knowledge. Although Weed's views did not materialise into an information system they influenced the development of future hospital information systems that took the medical process as a foundation. In the academic field the development of the HELP system by Homer Warner and Alan Pryor at the University of Utah was a seminal example of this approach. The HELP (Health Evaluation through Logic Processing) system was built with the idea of using patient data and medical knowledge ('*logic processing*') to support clinical decision making.

In the practice area the development of the TDS system (formerly Technicon system) proved to be of great importance, providing support for medical and nursing care based on patient care transactions. The system was designed in a such a way that physicians or nurses needed no technical knowledge to use a computer terminal and could use the terminology they used in daily practice. The system used the principle of what is now called user-centred design.

The third phase, of knowledge applications, saw the emergence of knowledge-based systems. This development was driven by research in artificial intelligence (AI) in the 1950s and 1960s and the fact that uncertainty problems in medicine were an excellent test bed for exploring ideas in AI research. Uncertainty problems were recognised as intrinsic to medicine through the important work in clinical decision analysis using probability theory and Bayesian statistics by Ledley & Lusted in the 1950s (Ledley & Lusted 1959). It is only in the last decade that attention has shifted to important practical problems in medicine.

We are now witnessing a merging of the three phases. For example, important progress is being made in the analysis of signals and the diagnostic interpretation of them by means of AI techniques. Information systems are embedded with intelligence so that they not only present information but also issue alerts when certain values of patient parameters are reached. These values are automatically derived from the medical condition of that particular patient. The above-mentioned HELP system is a good example of this merging, as is the connection of physiological monitoring equipment with information systems.

Definitions of medical informatics reflect this merging of the three phases, and also recognise the shift from concentration on automated machines to the nature of medical data, information and knowledge itself. Greenes & Shortliffe (1990) define medical informatics as 'the field concerned with the cognitive, information processing, and communication tasks of medical practice, education and research, including the information science and technology to support these tasks'. This definition shows clearly that the practice of medicine is the starting point but that automated machines can be the object of study when they are pertinent to medical practice. Greenes & Shortliffe's definition has undergone criticism because it suggests that medical informatics will generate new professionals who will claim that they are trained in information management and know how to interpret medical data (Anon 1990). The fear is expressed that physicians who are not fully computer literate will be deprived of direct access to medical data.

Greenes & Shortliffe also state that the emergence of the new discipline finds its roots in the explosion of medical knowledge, an explosion so great that no individual physician is able to comprehend it all. Thus one can observe that in the US the National Library of Medicine is taking the lead in developing the discipline by funding most of the research. More recently Shortliffe (1991) has expanded the definition to include medical problem solving, thus incorporating the results of research in clinical decision support.

Other authors offer definitions that characterise what the field is dealing with, rather than what it actually is. Reichertz for example described the application areas of medical informatics as 'information acquisition, information retrieval, information evaluation, information storage, flow control and man-machine interface', emphasising the technological aspects of medical informatics (Möhr 1989). In that respect he considered medical informatics as an applied science that should be judged against its practical achievements. Braude (1987) states that medical informatics is 'the application of computer science to the field of medicine', but this definition simply makes computer science and informatics identical.

TOWARDS A FOUNDING PRINCIPLE OF NURSING INFORMATICS

Van Bemmel (1984), however, proposes a clear definition by focusing on information processing and communication irrespective of the means. He writes that 'medical informatics comprises the

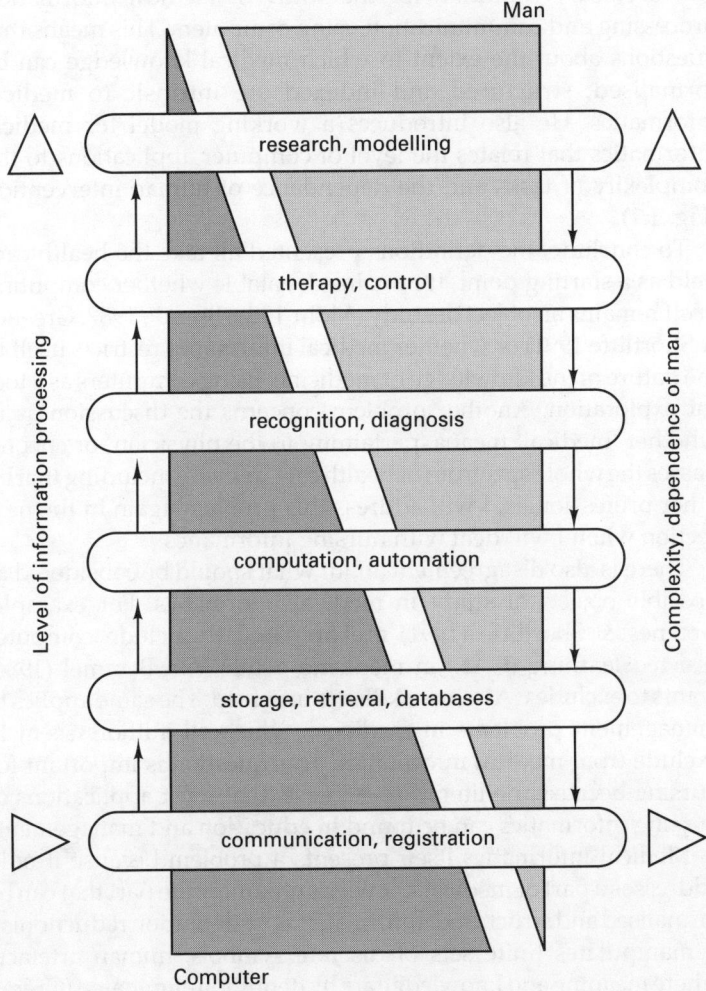

Figure 1.1 A working model of schematic representation for the ordering of computer applications in medicine. The model consists of six levels of complexity, where, from bottom to top, the computer influence as an autonomous machine decreases and human influence and intervention increases (after Van Bemmel 1984).

theoretical and practical aspects of information processing and communication, based on knowledge and experience derived from processes in medicine and health care'. He makes clear that a thorough understanding of processes in medicine and health care is a necessary condition for the study of medical information processing and communication using computers. This means that questions about the extent to which medical knowledge can be formalised, structured and indexed are intrinsic to medical informatics. He also introduces a working model for medical informatics that relates the level of computer applications to the complexity of tasks and the dependence of human intervention (Fig. 1.1).

To conclude, the definitions presented all take the health care field as a starting point. It remains debatable whether computing itself remains an object of study (Möhr 1989, Braude 1987, Greenes & Shortliffe 1991) or whether medical informatics restricts itself to the nature of the knowledge of medicine, using computers as a tool for exploration. Another problem concerns the discussion as to whether 'medical' means 'pertaining to the physician' or encompasses the whole spectrum of health care delivery including that by other professionals. I will address this problem again in the next section when I will deal with nursing informatics.

There is also disagreement about what should be considered as possible objects of study in medical informatics. For example, Greenes & Shortliffe (1991) are prepared to include computer assisted learning (CAL) in medicine, while Van Bemmel (1984) wants to exclude CAL since skills are involved. The same applies to management problems in medicine, which all authors seem to exclude from medical informatics. This question is important for nursing because the literature suggests that most applications of nursing informatics can be found in education and management.

Medical informatics itself presents a problem because it only addresses a part of medical knowledge, namely the part that can be formalised and structured. Informatics is by definition reductionist; it manipulates finite sets of discrete symbols, human artefacts where meaning and knowledge are by definition eliminated (Grémy 1989). According to Grémy this conflicts with a humanistic approach in medicine. His concerns reflect the more general uneasiness that the effect of modern technology on health care carries the risk of dehumanising the patient and reducing him to an object deprived of meaning.

We can conclude that all definitions presented take health care delivery as a starting point. Disagreement exists about the role of computer technology and the scope of medical informatics. Möhr et al (1989) sigh 'that the establishment of a common concept of medical informatics is still beyond the horizon'.

NURSING INFORMATICS

Real interest in the use of computers in nursing started when Bitzer (1966) described how she used the PLATO system (one of the earliest authoring systems, implemented on a mainframe computer) to develop a program for computer-assisted learning.

It is interesting to note that awareness of the possible benefits of automation originated at about the same time as the pioneering work in medical informatics. An editorial in *Nursing Forum* (Anon 1962) gives a philosophical overview, asking 'what will automation mean for nursing and nurses?' and pleading with nurses not to adopt nursing's historic weapon against change, passive resistance, which 'could lead us to professional suicide', but to think positively and plan now for the 'automated world we are destined to live in'.

Generally the development of nursing informatics parallels that of medical informatics. The emphasis of the role of the computer is on the savings that can be achieved in the area of administrative work in nursing (Table 1.1) and for that reason administrative applications received considerable attention. In some cases nursing was involved at an early stage in the development of information systems. The development of the TDS system in the 1970s was a good example of such involvement.

Unlike medicine, nursing considers the use of computers to be a vehicle to advance the status of the profession. This fact is closely related to the emergence of nursing as a professional discipline with an academic recognition. One sees that nursing puts much effort into developing 'nursing theories' expressing views about human behaviour, the attitude of humans towards health and disease and the role of nursing in the processes of recovery or stabilisation (Fawcett 1989). Many of these theories have been poorly researched in practice and often include views about human behaviour based on outdated theories such as Maslow's hierarchy of needs. However, it must be recognised that a firm foundation of nursing is of utmost importance for the development of nursing applications.

Medicine has concentrated on well-defined application areas such as radiology and electrocardiography, but is now also facing the problem of clarification of the medical process in terms of complaints, findings, diagnosis, therapeutic goals, actions and evaluation. I will therefore turn to the nature of medical descriptions as described by Blois (1984) and see what is relevant for nursing.

Medicine deals with diseases in two ways. One approach is the nominalist account, in which a disease can be completely described in terms of its attributes and without any reference to patients. This procedure is commonly adopted when we deal with abstract ideas or concepts. The other approach is the attribute view of disease with the understanding that the attributes in this case are those of a particular patient. Here the emphasis is on the importance of the physician's detailed and systematic descriptions of his observations as he attempts to treat a particular individual's illness. The individual's condition when ill is distinguished by those attributes that represent deviations from his preceding healthy state. The latter approach has prompted the search for causes of these deviations, and here lies the core of science-based modern medicine.

The contrast between the nominal and the attribute views is well demonstrated by a comparison between psychiatry and clinical medicine. In psychiatry schizophrenia, for example, is described by attributes like 'shallow emotional response', 'restlessness', 'posturing', 'unpredictable behaviour', and so on. No single attribute would suffice for the diagnosis of this disorder. The description of

Table 1.2 Hierarchical levels of medical descriptions (after Blois 1984)

Level	Description
Level 0	Patient as a whole
Level -1	Major patient part e.g. chest, abdomen, head
Level -2	Physiological system e.g. cardiovascular system, respiratory system
Level -3	System part, or organ e.g. heart, major vessels, lungs
Level -4	Organ part, or tissue e.g. myocardium, bone marrow
Level -5	Cell e.g. epithelial cell, fibroblast, lymphocyte
Level -6	Cell part e.g. cell membrane, organelles, nucleus
Level -7	Macromolecule e.g. enzyme, structural protein, nucleic acid
Level -8	Micromolecule e.g. glucose, ascorbic acid
Level -9	Atoms or ions e.g. sodium, iron

The levels are indicated in descending order. The attributes at the top are usually of a generic nature and thus often ambiguous and/or fuzzy. In contrast, the attributes of the lowest level are mostly very well defined and can often be expressed in numerical values. Modern medicine is searching for attributes at a sufficiently low level that a description can be precise and actions more focused.

schizophrenia lies at a single, very high level where there is considerable fuzziness and ambiguity of reference, where explanations are at present unsatisfactory, where the sufficiency of attributes is not established and certainty in diagnosis is elusive.

In clinical medicine the cause of pneumonia has been well understood since the germ theory of disease became accepted. The diagnosis is focused on the identification of the infectious agent and the treatment is related to that identification. We can identify the disease for certain by the findings of an examination of the patient and from the cultures taken. The attributes relating to pneumonia are on a lower level (we know about the agent that causes the disease) than the attributes of schizophrenia.

According to Blois (1984) we can introduce hierarchical levels of medical descriptions which enable us to classify attributes (Table 1.2).

This classification makes it apparent that the attributes of schizophrenia which pertain to behaviour are to be found on the level where we describe the patient as a whole (level 0). In the case of pneumonia the attributes can be described in terms of symptoms (fever, level 0), affected physiological system (respiratory system, level - 2), causative agent (pneumococcus, level - 5). It now makes sense to make a distinction between illness and disease. Illnesses are high-level matters; patients go to the physician with complaints such as a headache or fatigue, but never (except perhaps for experienced diabetics) complaining of 'low blood sugar' but with no discernible symptoms. However, confronted with the patient's symptoms a physician will diagnose a disease that can be explained in terms of its low-level attributes.

In practice it is the low-level attributes that provide the strongest evidence for a diagnosis, but it is the high-level attributes that make patients describe themselves as ill. In the case of pneumonia, identifying infection by pneumococcus bacteria allows the physician to start a treatment with an antibiotic, rather than treating fever with blood letting. Thus we can see a reductionist bias: low-level explanations are so attractive because they can be reached from as few assumptions as possible (a principle known as Occam's Razor). The goal of the diagnostic process then is to achieve the most convincing explanation of the clinical findings in the light of existing knowledge.

How does nursing look at health problems? Even if nurses consider humans as whole (the holistic approach), health problems are related to distinguishable factors like disease, physical impairment, personal behaviour and attitudes and social circumstances, which must all be understood if they are to receive adequate nursing action. Nursing has therefore to rely on many sources of knowledge. Medical knowledge has already been assessed, but other sources are likely to be more difficult to describe, since their description will involve high-level attributes. Since nursing is dealing with high-level attributes it is faced with the problem that these attributes have little explanatory power. Nursing theories have arisen to tackle this problem but until now with very little success. When nursing deals with low-level activities such as medication or monitoring physiological signals this often results from the physician's orders.

The core concern of nursing is to deal with the health problems of patients and to identify actions that take into account the different sources of knowledge from which nurses draw. Co-ordinating the proper execution of these actions seems then to be a core activity. Nursing knowledge is related to specific knowledge to do with the identification of health problems and the provision of proper care, but nursing profits from an eclectic approach in which knowledge from a variety of sources will be integrated. Nursing uses its own language, but concepts of this language have to be explained in terms of existing knowledge.

Given the fact that an action is most effective when the low level attributes are known, the challenge for nursing is to research these attributes in the relevant non-medical domain. A proper definition of nursing diagnosis would follow that of medicine and could be phrased as the best possible assessment of a patient's health problems in the light of existing nursing knowledge.

A long-standing difficulty in nursing, as in medicine, has been the lack of a uniform nomenclature or coding for health problems. This lack forms a severe hindrance for the development of structured record-keeping systems and the computerisation of nursing information. Many problems have more than one name, and a single name can have different meanings. Naming is important because it can provide clues to relevant attributes, which then point to appropriate actions. In short, proper naming points to intrinsic nursing knowledge about that problem.

There are essentially three approaches towards classification or development of a standardised nomenclature. First, it is possible to establish a uniform naming system for health problems. Names are often based on the name of the individual who first described the problem (e.g. Parkinson's disease), but are shifting more towards using clues that give evidence about causation or point to a relation to another known problem (e.g. appendicitis). There is, however, no uniformity in the naming of health problems; names often arise out of circumstances and gradually an agreement develops as to the exact meaning of a name.

Using categories to group health problems one can assign numbers for the names, but these numbers have no numerical meaning since they are used for their cardinality. This approach is extremely popular with public health authorities and epidemiologists because the collecting and processing of public health data is greatly facilitated by the use of single names or numbers.

The most important example of this approach is the International Classification of Diseases (ICD) prepared under the auspices of the World Health Organization (WHO) (Health Care Financing Administration 1980). In the ICD coding scheme diseases are grouped in main categories such as locus or major physiological system or organs (head, extremities, cardiovascular system, etc.) and hierarchies that particularise diseases such as specifying the place of occurrence. Names are represented by three digit numbers. A fourth number is added as a refinement of the disease name. For example, acute myocardial infarction (410) can be refined by the addition of the location, such as anterolateral wall (410.0) or anterior wall (410.1). The current 9th version of the ICD will be replaced in a few years by the 10th version that will include nursing problems. The current work on a standardised nursing diagnosis classification by the North American Nursing Diagnosis Association (NANDA) is also an example of this approach.

Second, one can use attributes to provide for a classification. A particular instance of a health problem can then be described as the summation of a collection of these attributes. A good example of this approach is the use of Diagnostic and Statistical Manual for Mental Disorders (DSM-III-R) (Work Group to Revise DSM-III of the American Psychiatric Association 1987) which is now in its third revision. Attributes are grouped in categories (or 'axes') to provide for an adequate description of a particular mental problem in psychiatry. In nursing, the use of patient classification systems to assess the acuity of the patient and the necessary staffing is also an example of this approach.

Third, the last approach is to use a standard nomenclature of health problems that also states what each problem is. The first attempt at this approach is the Current Medical Information and Terminology (CMIT), that lists 3263 diseases alphabetically by their preferred name, provides an additional 5500 cross-referenced eponyms and synonyms and gives the major clinical, pathological, laboratory and radiological attributes that are regarded characteristic of each disease. The Unified Medical Language System (UMLS) initiated by the National Library of Medicine will provide a metathesaurus of concepts synthesised from existing sources like ICD-9, MeSH (Medical Subject Headings, used to classify biomedical literature), SNOMED (Systematised Nomenclature for Medicine, a classification scheme similar to that of DSM-III-R), DSM-III-R and other biomedical nomenclature and classification systems. By establishing links between the names and attributes of the existing systems, UMLS will provide for a complete lexicon of medical knowledge that can be accessed by computer.

Classification is an important step in the formalisation of nursing knowledge. Formalisation is so important because the use of automated information systems requires that knowledge is made completely explicit and represented in the form of symbols that can be manipulated. Naturally this raises the question of the extent to which nursing knowledge can be formalised. Other chapters in this book touch on possible answers to that problem.

Classification provides a means to use symbols to represent nursing knowledge. However, names and attributes are by themselves void of meaning. For example the name 'Parkinson's disease' does not by itself represent any knowledge. The name does not give any indication about its attributes. It is in the mind of the physician treating a health problem (the context) that this name will mean something and that the proper attributes will be recognised. It is to be hoped that the name will have the same meaning in the mind of another physician. The process of classification tries to achieve that shared understanding, giving rise to the development of a common body of knowledge for a particular problem area. The lexical approach contains knowledge because names and attributes are connected in a meaningful way.

We have briefly touched on the reasoning process in health care. Reasoning underlies decision making and is based on the available data and knowledge regarding a particular problem. Often data and knowledge are not complete and uncertainty enters the process. Because it is impossible to have complete knowledge about the health status of a person, uncertainty is intrinsic in the decision process.

Knowledge-based systems that support decision-making tasks model not only a particular problem area but also the uncertainties involved.

It can be concluded that there exists a discontinuity between the human information process and the use of a code to support the information process in a formalised system, whether it is paper- or computer-based. This discontinuity is not a concern of computer science. Following Blois, I would suggest that it is the task of nursing informatics to understand better and define the nursing information process in order that appropriate activities can be chosen for computerisation. Technical issues of computer science are only considered in the context of support for the information process and are relevant, for example, to identify the practical limits of computerised nursing information systems. But as technology changes over time new possibilities will arise that may now be considered impractical.

I would suggest that the engineering of nursing information systems is not an object of study in its own right within nursing informatics, but only when taken into account as part of the nursing information process. I am therefore tempted to reject those definitions that incorporate technological issues of medical computing as objects of study in their own right and that relate medical and nursing informatics to computer science.

With the help of the ordering scheme of Van Bemmel (Fig 1.1) it is now possible to define briefly a research agenda for nursing informatics. The scheme I will suggest could be imagined as an apartment building and the metaphor of entering the building through the ground floor indicates that the higher levels of informatics are firmly based on the lower levels, in a hierarchical relationship.

The level of communication and registration emphasises the aspects, for example, of communication and data entry in an information system and data logging in an intensive care unit. Research issues at this level comprise among others the design of interfaces between nurses and information systems that take into account the specific situation of working with a patient. The current interest in hand-held terminals and bed-side points of data entry makes this research very relevant. Nursing could benefit from knowledge in the field of human interface design, cognitive psychology and ergonomics.

At the level of database management research should focus on the development of standards for nursing data and knowledge, as discussed above. Current research is dealing with the Minimum Nursing Data Set (Werley et al 1991), standardised nursing diagnosis concepts through NANDA and the development of a lexicon and taxonomy for nursing interventions (Grobe 1990). More mundane subjects are the structure of the nursing or patient record and nursing component of health care information systems.

The level of computation and automation deals primarily with complicated calculating algorithms that are necessary for example to construct an image from absorption measurements of X-rays in computer tomography. This level bears little relevance for research in nursing informatics.

The next level of recognition and diagnosis is extremely relevant for nursing because at this level knowledge-based systems (or expert systems) come into play. Next to the necessity of well-defined nursing data and knowledge, research should focus on the reasoning process in nursing, the modelling of decision processes through the identification of inference rules and heuristics, and the question of the context in which knowledge-based systems can best be used. Currently knowledge-based systems perform well in narrowly defined knowledge areas. An example for nursing would be an expert system to assess the probability that a patient will develop bedsores.

The levels of therapy and control, and research and modelling are more distant from nursing. In the treatment of diabetes a portable pumping medication system is available that measures blood sugar levels and adapts the dispensing of insulin accordingly. Knowledge about the relationship between blood sugar levels and the administration of insulin is built into the machine. But it is extremely unlikely that a nurse will be replaced by a machine since the example refers to a well-defined task.

Some current research in biomedicine is based on explicit modelling of a research problem by mathematical equations. The investigation of physiological phenomena and pharmacokinetics that are characterised by low-level descriptions rely heavily on this approach. Opportunities for such approaches will not be found so easily in nursing, because of its concern with high-level descriptions.

The results of research have practical consequences for daily nursing activities. The development of nursing applications in clinical practice, administration and education has already benefited from work done in medical and nursing informatics and the engineering of information systems. Nursing and medicine may at times seem antagonistic to each other but both are concerned with providing services to the patient. The patient has a right to know that information processes are well taken care of. For both professions the patient's health problem is the same and close collaboration is necessary to provide for quality care. Therefore nursing and medical informatics are closely related.

REFERENCES

Anonymous 1962 Editorial: Untouched by human hands. Nursing Forum 1(2): 12–20
Anonymous 1990 Medical informatics. Lancet 335: 824–825
Bitzer M D 1966 Clinical nursing instruction via the PLATO simulated laboratory. Nursing Research 15: 144–150
Blois M S 1984 Information and medicine—the nature of medical descriptions. University of California Press, Berkeley
Blum B I 1986 Clinical information systems. Springer-Verlag, New York
Blum B I 1991 The software process for medical applications. In: Timmers T, Blum B I (eds) 1991 Software engineering in medical informatics. North-Holland, Amsterdam, pp 3–26
Braude R M 1987 Environmental and personal factors in secondary career choice of graduates of medical informatics training programs. Dissertation. University of Nebraska, Lincoln
Collen M F 1986 Origins of medical informatics. Western Journal of Medicine 145: 778–785
Fawcett J 1989 Analysis and evaluation of conceptual models of nursing. FA Davis Company, Philadelphia
Graves J R, Corcoran S 1989 The study of nursing informatics. Image 21: 227–231
Greenes R A, Shortliffe E H 1990 Medical informatics—an emerging academic discipline and institutional priority. Journal of the American Medical Association 263: 1114–1120
Grémy F 1989 Crisis of meaning and medical informatics education: a burden and/or a relief? Methods of Information in Medicine 28: 189–195
Grobe S J 1990 Nursing intervention and taxonomy study: language and classification methods. Advances in Nursing Science 13: 22–33
Health Care Financing Administration 1980 The international classification of diseases, 9th revision. Clinical Modification, US Department of Health and Human Services, Washington DC
Ledley R S, Lusted L B 1959 Reasoning foundations of medical diagnosis. Science 130: 9–21
Möhr J R 1989 Teaching medical informatics: teaching on the seams of disciplines, cultures, traditions. Methods of Information in Medicine 28: 273–280
Möhr J R, Protti D J, Salamon R 1989 Medical informatics and education (editorial). Methods of Information in Medicine 28: 187–188
Shortliffe E H 1991 Medical informatics and clinical decision making—the science and the pragmatics. Medical Decision Making 11 (suppl): S2–S14
Van Bemmel J H 1984 The structure of medical informatics. Medical Informatics 9: 175–180

Weed L L 1969 Medical records, medical education and patient care. The Press of Case Western Reserve University, Cleveland

Werley H H, Devine E C, Zorn C R, Ryan P, Westra B L 1991 The nursing minimum data set: abstraction tool for standardised, comparable, essential data. American Journal of Public Health 81: 421–426

Work Group to Revise DSM-III of the American Psychiatric Association 1987 Diagnostic and Statistical Manual of Mental Disorders, 3rd edition (revised). American Psychiatric Association, Washington DC

2

From village to big city: nursing informatics

P. Verduin   P. Epping

Introduction	Co-operation with the world
The society metaphor	Co-operation with each other
Some considerations	Justification of a choice
Guiding concepts	A perspective on communication
Choice	Conclusion

INTRODUCTION

In this chapter we would like to highlight some basic principles of nursing informatics based on recent developments in the philosophy of science. This endeavour will not be a simple one within the environment of a hard science like informatics.

Because there is no agreement with regard to founding principles in discussions about nursing informatics (although see also Chapter 1 by Jos Aarts),we intend to give some ideas or guidelines, more with the intention of stimulating reflection and imagination than in the hope of giving answers or suggesting behaviour. Some considerations may be important for the way in which informatics is used in nursing and how it is experienced and perceived: as a challenging but helpful development, as a threat, or as both challenge and threat. We will try to address the problem of what is good for nursing informatics and what is not good.

The approach will be from outside nursing informatics and actually is a translation of ideas developed in the philosophy of science.

THE SOCIETY METAPHOR

The following considerations are structured by the use of a metaphor to clarify some of the possibilities and problems of our postmodern era. Within this metaphor we prefer to see our modern era as a 'village' and the post-modern era as a 'city' (de Vries 1991).

De Vries asked himself how we can have a mental image of a human society in which technological culture is so very important.

He paints a picture of a big city, with many people on pavements, walking past illuminated shop windows with displays of things we have not seen being made: French cheese, beer from Belgium or a pocket-calculator from Japan. There are many cars moving fast in different directions, the noise of underground trains and aeroplanes, foreign papers, illuminated advertising and so on.

If we paint human society in terms of a village, rather than a big city, we see many differences: physical space and social space are much smaller, even fenced in. The village green is a geographical and social centre. Only a few houses away is the end of the village and the beginning of the farm-lands. The neighbouring village is an 'other' village with its own centre and own mores.

Social roles in the village are clear to everyone: the teacher, baker or police officer are known as people. Even if they are not at work they will be known as baker or teacher, with the expectations that accompany their function.

In village life, time has a shared meaning: eating at 6 p.m., turning out the light at 10.30 p.m.; deviations will soon be noticed and discussed.

On the other hand, life in the city is an amalgamation of connections and networks. Close-by and far-away have a different meaning. The railway connects different cities supplying products from far away, but separates the city into two parts whose inhabitants will hardly ever see each other.

In the city people are not together in a given social space, with explicit common values, periodically renewed in significant rituals from which the self and common feeling is derived, as they are in the village.

Using these ideas, of the 'village' and the 'big city', we will try to clarify some of the principles that are developing in nursing informatics.

SOME CONSIDERATIONS

Using the metaphor of the village and the city is risky because it might lead to unwanted conclusions. Transforming our society to a post-modern, technological society, from village to city, from 'Gemeinschaft' to 'Gesellschaft', could be seen as estranging, because it often seems that in the old days everything was better. On this basis people might argue that we don't need informatics at all! However, that would be wanting to live in the past, striving after established structures that are guidelines for our lives. We will call this the 'romantic' attitude, romantic because in this attitude lost feelings must be rebuilt, and because it is accompanied by some sadness or even fatalistic feelings. We do not want this chapter to descend into nostalgia.

A second risk of our post-modern, technological society and the presence of nursing informatics (in terms of the big city metaphor) is that it may lead to a false optimism, and a belief that technology can solve all our problems—an optimism that hardly differs from the romantic attitude.

A characteristic of this romantic view is the belief that it is possible to create uniform procedures, agreements and schemes by which all problems can be solved. The answer can always be given by a theory, paradigm, or meta-paradigm, or by a program that helps us solve every nursing problem. This optimism is very like the romantic attitude because it has its roots in the same problem: that of looking at the big city from the perspective of the village. We will try to make sure that our discourse does not fall into a similar error.

Thirdly, we must not become negative or indifferent to the amazing achievements of modern technology that make our lives more pleasant. Supposing we had to write this article without a computer, or manage stock-control without a computer, or produce the duty roster without a computer. We must not throw the baby out with the bath water.

GUIDING CONCEPTS

With regard to nursing practice we see two principal guidelines. The first involves a humanistic approach in which reasoning processes, personal involvement and responsibility are the points of reference for making decisions. We are not speaking here of a complete picture, but of an elusive game of heterogeneous strengths in which we are involved and in which we are constituent in a contingent way.

These heterogeneous strengths are:

- personal values, thoughts and expectations being generated and being given meaning in conjunction with
- rules with regard to time and space, expectations, requirements, and procedures, whether or not they have a legal status. This game of individual and collective strengths can be seen in relation to another strength, namely:

- the impact of the material environment: the presence of information machines and software, and the behaviour or actions which it invites or imposes.

In our view this informatics environment is explicitly joined with these three elements; as a 'praxis', a way in which people can engage with it.

The second way of guiding this praxis is by reference to the village model. Earlier in the chapter we discussed the romantic and optimistic views. These views are quite opposite to the humanistic approach: in both of them the big city is being perceived from the perspective of a village.

The optimistic view is characterised by established frameworks, in which co-operation has been fixed. This view can easily develop into a technocratic way of thinking, with decisions being made by a small group of so-called experts. People expect that these experts can justify their decisions by reference to the hard scientific opinions in which they are the experts. Some experts indeed claim that their assertions or decisions can be confirmed in that way and that they can fulfil such expectations.

In the romantic view there are the same fundamental assumptions: there is the belief that in the past there were established frameworks, and the expectation is that with some endeavour we can return to these frameworks and manage without the help of the experts and their methods.

The difference between the two ways of guiding is that the village mentality supposes that there is an ongoing, independent objective framework of laws and regularities within which we can operate. This assumption denies the contingency of the first (humanistic) approach. In the big city model we can only achieve a relative stability by reference to fundamental principles, rather than absolute rules or laws. In the big city model of the postmodern, technological society, instability and unpredictability are defining characteristics.

Because of this unpredictability there is a danger that we may lose control. In our society we can prevent this by making agreements, rules and, particularly with regard to informatics, standards. Often this has been achieved by the development of conventions which guarantee a relative stability and continuity, without losing sight of contingency.

CHOICE

The next question is: why do we want to see our society as a post-modern, technological society, described in terms of a big city rather than the village metaphor? There are different sources from which we can underpin our idea of post-modern technological culture, and nursing informatics within it, and from which we can see it as a contingent, dynamic society. For this purpose we can look to a discussion of our co-operation with the world and with each other.

CO-OPERATION WITH THE WORLD

Science, and technology derived from science, have played an important role for a very long time in our dealings with the problems of our material society. Thinking about science has brought us many quite new ideas, ideas that are irrationally denied in many situations.

The work of Merleau-Ponty (1945) has revolutionised contemporary images of science. His analysis of perception called into question the whole idea of an established world. In his view, perception brings us into contact with things, and gives the opportunity for the opening, the passage to the things. Perception is an experience confirmed by subsequent experiences existing as a coherent whole. This suggests that there is an absolute perspective on an object that includes the entire truth.

But confirmation never is absolute. It results in a never ending process of perception, which is vague in the beginning but which gets clearer during the process. If there were such a thing as an absolute perspective it would mean that there would be no point of view to which we could relate our perception. This in turn would mean that there is no observer and so there can be no big city. But perception is the experience of our concrete existence, the basis of our process of knowledge building.

With regard to nursing informatics, we can state that there is no picture of the whole, and in fact nobody knows all the aspects of nursing informatics. Different perspectives are possible: rich, broad, one-sided, appropriate, inappropriate, just, unjust and so on. These perspectives need not be a threat to the rational development of nursing informatics: in fact they are prerequisites.

CO-OPERATION WITH EACH OTHER

There are many beautiful things surrounding us, but we must also acknowledge the existence of evil, oppression and cruelty. These occur in wars, prisons and concentration camps, in the name of fundamentalist theories, in the name of the true belief, the only program that can help your organisation. Of course there are no murderers in nursing informatics, but oppression by structural power is possible.

In the pursuit of economic goals at the beginning of this century scientific management or Taylorism was developed. It could be argued that Taylorism is not possible within informatics: employees principally need more scope to give their best, they have to have more responsibility and they have to be flexible. On the other hand informatics is a perfect tool with which management can control employees. Their identity cards betray all their movements in the organisation. A panoptical control is possible. In a modern variation of Taylorism it is possible to develop programs that control people's work, forcing them to work according to what is in the program, under the direction of the program.

Is this kind of control a bad thing? This question cannot be answered easily. It depends on the answers to questions such as: 'to what purpose?' or 'in whose interest?'. This lies at the very heart of our discussion. If we are to ask questions and give answers regarding the meaning and justice of procedures, theories, acts and rules we must have living, feeling and tangible people. Their judgement, imagination and ability to give meaning cannot be formalised because of the dynamic character of perception and interpretation. We want to see formalisation as a provisional standardisation of the full act, not as an expedient means of considering the complex dynamic character of a situation in order to make a temporary gain in time or efficiency. We can regard conventions, rules and expectations about the way we co-operate with each other generally as formalisation. The value of this is obvious: it gives at least a minimal relative stability and continuity necessary in our highly dynamic society. Formalisation at this level can be seen as providing bearing points. And just here, in what we might call the *life-world*, including our ability to interpret and to justify those interpretations, we find it possible to criticise and influence the systems, organisations, and institutions that may be created.

JUSTIFICATION OF A CHOICE

Having considered the question of why the big city metaphor fits better than the idea of the village as a metaphor of our modern society, an important step in our discussion is to address the question of why the romantic vision is so bad or why the post-modern 'big city' idea is so good in guiding the relationship between nursing and informatics.

The romantic vision brings with it the real danger that we may fall into apathy or indifference about our situation. The idea also could fail if there is an unrealistic belief that 'everything is possible'. Depression and despair lie in wait and there is a real chance that we will not be able to do anything. There are similar dangers with the romantic view, because responsibility simply has been handed over to the experts.

The normative point of view is directly derived from what we have already stated above: *it is based on assumptions about the contingent and complex character of our society and within our society the unpredictable game of heterogeneous strengths, and our view of health services, including nursing informatics, as a 'big city phenomenon'. We are trying in an open way to create an interest group, using our human capacity to achieve rational agreement about the problems and questions concerning nursing informatics.* If we are to achieve this agreement we need a broad view on rationalism, towards which important contributions have already been made by Habermas (1981, 1985, 1988) and Kunneman (1986, 1989).

A PERSPECTIVE ON COMMUNICATION

Distinctive within this approach by Kunneman, derived from the work of Habermas, is that all action is communication. If we are to say anything valid about an action we must consider all of the following:

1. *the cognitive–instrumental reality domain* (for instance the techniques of hardware and software, the skills to handle it, financial and educational requirements)
2. *the aesthetic–expressive reality domain* (for instance that which you want to achieve personally, wishes, needs, talents and limitations in certain situations)

3. *the moral–practical reality domain* (relationships in which people co-operate, expectations, goals and conventions that make possible stability and continuity in co-operation).

Between these three domains there is a connection (see Fig. 2.1), but for the purpose of analysis there can be a relative independence. This is important because now we are able to prevent indifference, relativism, etc.

In relation to these domains we can distinguish the following criteria:

- *Efficiency* is the measure of the quality of technical or instrumental developments. These developments lead to successful acts being achieved in the area of the cognitive–instrumental domain. These successful acts must be judged in terms of the existing concepts within this domain.
- Using the criterion *authenticity* we can say something about personal involvement, about feelings related to values and the integrity of personal actions. Using this criterion we can evaluate the aesthetic–expressive reality domain.
- *Justice*: Evaluation of the humanity or justice of a proposal, argument or act is the critical measure of the moral–practical reality domain.

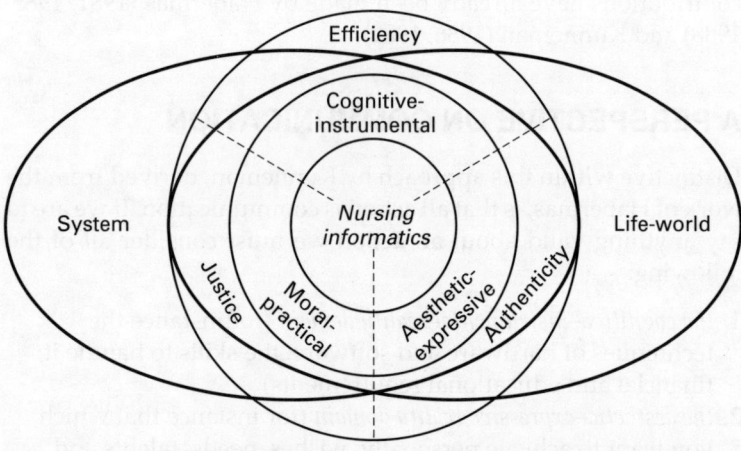

Figure 2.1 An approach to nursing informatics as a space of interference between life-world and system.

Of course there are many problems to be overcome, especially regarding the definitions of nursing informatics. It will also be very difficult to argue claims regarding humanity and justice. Evaluation of normative arguments in terms of their tenability and relevance distinguishes them from descriptive assertions.

There is a tendency for this difference to be forgotten and for all assertions to be treated as if they were descriptive. If this happens there is no relative distinction between the cognitive–instrumental and moral–practical reality domains, and technical–instrumental interpretations, and so proposals become immune from criticism regarding their normative implications.

Now we must try to join the nursing context to information technology. Besides the questions already mentioned this endeavour directly refers to the question 'what should be the content of nursing and what should be our image and identity?'

Regarding nursing informatics we must be wary of indifference on the one hand and high expectations on the other: for example indifference to mistakes in software, or high expectations in the case of expert systems. Expert systems should bring us enormous benefits; the skill of an expert put into a computer, possibly reducing a post-modern broad rationalism into a one-sided modern cognitive instrumental rationality.

In that model we also want to consider the area of the nursing data which can be collected regarding the broad perspective (cognitive–instrumental, aesthetic–expressive and moral–practical domains). If we consider the Nursing Information Management model constructed by Graves & Corcoran (1989) we can see that this is very close to the cognitive–instrumental domain. Goossen (1992) has expanded this model, making it possible to include the aesthetic–expressive domain. However, there is still no relationship with the moral–practical domain; this could perhaps be linked to the decision part of the model. If we have to emphasise just the technical part (cognitive–instrumental domain) then we are very conscious of it. But now, we know what is missing and what therefore must somehow be added.

In the communication–theoretical perspective we first consider nursing informatics as a subsystem of material reproduction of society in which we recognise analogous conventions. In this study we state that nursing informatics cannot be considered as a description of a (sub)system, but, discussed as a communicative problem, nursing informatics can be seen as an interference phenomenon between life-world and system. In our approach to this problem we must be careful not to allow ourselves to be pushed aside by system imperatives; we must discuss system developments by putting them in a broad rational perspective. Specific life-world needs occur in the interference space. Now, both system imperatives and life-world needs can be discussed using the criteria discussed above. With the help of communicative rationality we can, according to Habermas, not only indicate forms of structural violence, but also strive for a reconciliation between system and life-world, a reconciliation in which system and life-world are so attuned that system imperatives can get more feedback from life-world needs instead of predominantly or exclusively from technical limitations and economical objectives (Verduin, 1992).

CONCLUSION

In this paper an attempt has been made to put nursing informatics into a philosophical perspective. In a metaphorical description of our post-modern era we have chosen a dynamic model, which can be compared to a big city.

Nursing and nursing informatics are phenomena always in motion and cannot be caught in models. These constraints can be exposed by putting developments into the perspective of a broad rationality. To obtain insight into the information process in nursing, help can be found in the analysis of nursing language. The methods for such analysis have been presented and worked out by Habermas (1988) and Kunneman (1989).

We want to invite all nurses to discuss the developments in nursing informatics, using the ideas we have presented here. The multiform of the broad perspective is a prerequisite for the responsible development and guiding of nursing informatics.

REFERENCES

de Vries 1991 Hoe te leven in een technologische cultuur. Krisis 45: 34–46
Goossen W 1992 Verpleegkundige informatiekunde. Een noodzakelijke intermediair tussen verpleegkunde en informatica? Tijdschift voor Medische Informatica 21: 9–17
Graves J R, Corcoran S 1989 The study of nursing informatics. Image 21: 227–231
Grémy F 1989 Crisis of meaning in medical informatics education: a burden and/or relief? Methods of Information in Medicine 28: 189–195
Habermas J 1981 Theorie des kommunikativen Handelns, part I en II. Suhrkamp Verlag, Frankfurt am Main

Habermas J 1985 Die neue Unübersichtlichkeit. Suhrkamp Verlag, Frankfurt am Main

Habermas J 1988 Nachmetaphysisches Denken: Philosophische Aufsätze. Suhrkamp Verlag, Frankfurt am Main

Kunneman H 1986 De waarheidstrechter, een communicatie-theoretisch perspectief op wetenschap en samenleving. Boom, Meppel/Amsterdam

Kunneman H 1989 'Een model voor communicatie-theoretisch inter-ferentie-onderzoek'. In: Kunneman H (ed) Systeemgeweld en schijncommunicatie, Cahiers Communicatietheorie & praktijk 1. Faculteit der Wijsbegeerte, Universiteit van Amsterdam

Merleau-Ponty M 1945 Phénoménologie de la perception. Gallimard, Paris

Verduin P J M 1992 Het verdachte lichaam. De rationaliteit van het (para)medisch handelen bij somatisatiestoornissen in communicatie-theoretische perspectief. Thesis Publishers, Amsterdam

3

Formalising nursing knowledge

M. Theobald

Introduction
The beginnings of the problem
The phenomenon of nursing
   Introduction
   The function of nursing
   Example, Example, Example

The purpose of nursing
Report on a research activity
   Discussion
Types of knowledge
Conclusion

> 'Knowledge is of what cannot be otherwise'
>   Aristotle

INTRODUCTION

Why and how should we formalise nursing knowledge? This problem was presented to us during the first European Nursing Informatics Summer School, and for an entire week a group of people attempted to find an answer. The group included people from the United Kingdom, Belgium, Holland, Germany and Eire so it is perhaps not surprising that in the absence of a common language we struggled, through our shared nursing culture, to discover a common nursing language. As with so many complex issues the benefits lay as much in the exploration as in the findings.

Why was our task so difficult? Isn't nursing, after all, at least a common starting point? This chapter will be concerned with some of the difficulties inherent in the problem and in the reality of an under-researched area.

THE BEGINNINGS OF THE PROBLEM

If we are to achieve a common nursing language, nursing knowledge must be formalised. By this I mean that the language used in nursing must be identified and acknowledged so that we can be sure that it means the same to whoever uses it and whenever it is used. There are many difficulties inherent in attempting to find a common language in any situation and the following exercise (introduced by Dr Alan Hyslop at the Summer School) will illustrate the point. You might wish to try this yourself.

Two people can use this exercise to demonstrate the problem satisfactorily, although a group of up to twelve would offer more opportunities to explore the complexities. If two people are taking part each person is required to introduce him or herself to the other in whatever way he or she chooses. In doing this each participant must write a list of items which would represent the knowledge he or she would like to have about the other person in order to know them in a way which was satisfactory to both.

Upon completion of this task the lists are simply compared. If a larger group is taking part, one member may be chosen to supply his or her list as a baseline against which all others may be compared. Items from the other lists may be added to the base list, providing there is general agreement as to the importance of its inclusion. The final agreed list is then scored according to the merit of each item, allowing the items to be ranked in order of importance. The first five items can be agreed to be the most valued. Half the group may then be asked to reconsider the language used to express the knowledge people believed it was important to have, bearing in mind that the initial language used was the property of only one of the group. This proves to have difficult consequences later on, because the language chosen by this half of the group is likely to be different to the language used by the other half. If you had any doubts about the difficulties of finding a common nursing language, the difficulties arising from use of what is already considered a common language, English, will remove them.

Let us continue with our attempts to find a common nursing language. It seems to me that such nursing language when used, whether prescriptively or descriptively, presupposes the existence of nursing knowledge. And herein lies our problem. What is this knowledge? Or put another way, what is the nature of nursing knowledge? If there are verifiable answers to these questions then it must be that expert knowledge can be made explicit. Knowledge can be reduced to elements, generalisable reasoning strategies exist and, perhaps, action is the result of rational and logical procedures. Or is this true only insofar as the determining mode is a rationalist one?

The phenomenologists would, of course, argue quite differently. But what is the phenomenon of nursing? It might be appropriate to consider why the problem requires some urgent attention and what the issue is in relation to nursing informatics. Consider, therefore, the following. The recent introduction in the United Kingdom of the Resource Management Initiative (RMI) offers evidence that the language of reflection and its requirements of the skills of analysis have outstripped the practical reality. RMI has raised the questions of what health care professionals do and of what they achieve in relation to cost. Nurses have been involved in the introduction of nursing information systems, which are necessary to RMI, and some have been asked to write operational requirements for computer programmes.

It has become quite evident that nurses do not find it easy to formalise nursing knowledge, and that the skills of analysis are underdeveloped. Groups of nurses have been gathered together in order to determine what nursing is in order to identify the information to be collected which will enable effective and efficient nursing planning, and enable effective and efficient nursing practice to be carried out. The question 'What is nursing?' might appear simple enough on the face of it, and yet when it is put to nurses they tend to exhibit signs of anxiety.

Why should this be so? Partly, this is because the question sounds so simple that it appears to require a ready response. And yet a simple 'Nursing is what nurses practice' in this instance will not do. Indeed, if pressed one discovers that the questioner is not satisfied even if offered one of several phenomenological accounts. This, I suspect, is because he does not want to hear about what is the essence of nursing nor about what nurses do. He really wants to hear about what nurses know: the nature of nursing knowledge. Indeed, the formalization of that nursing knowledge which is necessary to write an operational requirement for a computerised information system concerns itself with the nature of nursing knowledge as it differs from medical knowledge or that of any other health care professional. But how do we formalise this knowledge?

In summary, it seems that there is an inability to identify nursing knowledge or indeed to clarify the difference between that knowledge which is applied to nursing practice and that which is deduced from it. There is uncertainty as to the nature of that knowledge which is created through professional practice.

THE PHENOMENON OF NURSING

Introduction

There are two particular issues in relation to nursing which need to be unravelled. One refers to purpose whilst the other refers to function. Very often nursing is described in terms of functions, by which I mean that nurses concern themselves with identifying exactly what they do and what actions they take in the course of a day. These functions they argue are embedded in the role of the nurse and offer professional parameters which undeniably belong to the nurse. Let us explore this.

The function of nursing

There are some difficulties attached to the problem of function when attempting to determine what is nursing. For example, nurses make beds. Does the act of making a bed make a nurse? Clearly not, as many people who would not describe themselves as nurses also make beds. What of making the bed of a sick person whilst that person is still in the bed? Again many carers find themselves required to perform such a function, but do not describe themselves as nurses nor are they legally able to do so.

The argument might then proceed towards identifying more complex skills, such as the administration of a drug by injection. This is something which nurses do, but so increasingly do ambulance drivers, other skilled paramedics, and many patients and their families. So what other functions might we consider? What of the functions required of a nurse in life-threatening situations? For example cardio-pulmonary resuscitation? It is true that nurses do perform such functions, usually in hospital settings, but so do many others, such as paramedics, first-aiders and swimming instructors. Indeed, some would argue that it is the duty of all citizens to learn such a skill in order to fulfil their public duty towards other citizens.

I believe that rather more complex skills lie in the arena of interpersonal interactions, such as breaking bad news, or spending time with a dying person in order to make the time available of value to that individual. But it has to be said yet again that these functions, however well or badly performed, are performed by other persons also, whether such persons be professionals or not. It might be possible to examine the notion of performance criteria in order to decide whether a highly skilled performance is characteristic of the work of a professional while a low level performance characterises the non-professional performance. This does present difficulties of its own, as some lay persons, because of experience in an intense situation, would score more highly than a qualified nurse in a given area of skill.

Example

Consider this description of a man suffering from Parkinson's disease. The man, aged 66 years, lived at home with his wife. Most sufferers do live at home with little or no professional support. Community nursing services were not provided, nor were they requested. It was considered to be the family's business. The man grew increasingly frail and forgetful, and to an onlooker it appeared that although he was constantly in need he was unable to express his needs either quickly enough or intelligibly enough for them to respond effectively.

His needs were met, however, very effectively, because his wife had learned to interpret his every move and expression. Certain movements were an indication that he was uncomfortable, but able to do something about it himself without help. Other movements indicated that he needed help to move from his chair. To the onlooker the difference between the two signals was almost indistinguishable. However, observation and experience had enabled his wife to interpret his body language in a way which others were unable to achieve.

What does experience in this context really mean? Facial expressions in a person suffering from Parkinson's disease are much reduced as the disease progresses, but in this case slight movements could be decoded by the patient's wife, who then acted accordingly. The wife's performance could be seen as that of a highly skilled performer, although she was not a nurse. This is not to say that a nurse might not become as skilled given the opportunity: the point is that such a skilled performance does not require a nurse.

And yet nursing does exist. The designation 'nurse' is a legal entity. Nursing is a self-regulating profession. The United Kingdom Central Council maintains a register of those entitled to call themselves nurses and charges the four national Boards with approving the education programmes which allow admission to this register and use of the title 'nurse'. Nurses are accountable for their practice in law.

The inability to identify professional characteristics by function alone does not apply only to nurses. All health care professionals suffer the same problem. And it is a problem, not least because many nurses continue in the hope that one day someone will define all professions in such a functional way and thus remove them and all other health care professionals from the vulnerable position in which they find themselves today of having to justify their existence.

Example

I spent an afternoon with a group of senior nursing colleagues who were trying to determine the different activities which could be performed by a health care support worker rather than a nurse. 60% of those present believed that it was possible to identify the differences between nurses and support workers in terms of functions. But not even the 60% could agree on which functions properly belonged to which group.

In today's world of multi-skilling and patient-focused hospitals there are those who might say that it is not only impossible but also undesirable to identify professional parameters by function. In the name of cost efficiency and cost containment the Secretary of State for Health and her ministers wish to see fewer professionals, each with a broader skill base. This is seen as a threat by professionals, who attempt to argue that retention of traditional barriers is in the patient's best interest (an example perhaps of Bernard Shaw's view that professionalism is a conspiracy against the laity?). And yet nursing does exist.

Example

A recent observation of a person suffering from stomach cancer served as a reminder that no matter what the confusion in the minds of nurses and managers about the role of the nurse, patients and clients know the worth of nursing, and for them nursing has meaning. This patient was also being cared for at home. The diagnosis of stomach cancer was made and the patient was informed by his general practitioner. At first surgery was suggested, but within 2 weeks of the initial diagnosis the patient and his family were told that surgery was not possible as the disease was too extensive and too advanced for an operation to offer any benefit.

The family supported each other in coming to terms with the future and at the end of the third week a nurse was assigned to their case. Five weeks later the patient had become very frail, his appetite was poor and the morphine prescribed to relieve his pain made him drowsy and forgetful. He vomited occasionally and his legs became swollen. All of this caused considerable distress to his wife who was also getting less sleep than she needed. When asked how she was coping she replied, 'I'll be all right, thank you, because nurse is coming in the morning.'

The trust expressed in those few words served as a timely reminder that whatever nursing is, it must be preserved. The wife did not want her husband in hospital. She was not asking the nurse to do anything in the functional sense, but she did need to ask her questions about the drugs her husband was taking, their purpose and any side-effects. She wanted to know that what she was doing was contributing to her husband's care and that she was not the cause of his worsening condition. She needed the nurse as a knowledgeable, objective outsider.

Having looked at the functions of nursing and worried about the fact that such functions are clearly not exclusive to nurses, the question must be asked, is the point really to identify exclusivity? Is it not enough to acknowledge that, in part, professional nursing aims to reach the same standards of loving care which are reached by a close relative when caring for a member of his or her family? Professional nursing requires duty rather than love. It is driven by a respect for persons, whether such persons be likeable or not and whether by their deeds they be deserving or not. It concerns itself with the delivery of excellent care to unknown persons rather than to loved ones, and with partiality towards no-one.

THE PURPOSE OF NURSING

The Concise Oxford Dictionary suggests that function 'is the mode of action or activity by which a thing fulfils its purpose', and purpose, it suggests, is 'the object to be obtained, the thing intended'. Function, in other words, concerns itself with what is done, whereas purpose concerns itself with why it is done. Function sits well with performance, purpose with illumination. Health service economists are forever searching for evidence of value for money, and rightly so. They ask questions such as, 'Why is it necessary to have a nurse to make beds, give bedpans, wash people or feed them? These are not high-level skills and they are easy to learn. You could train the average intelligent Brownie in those activities over a weekend.'

On the basis of the tasks alone it would be hard to disagree, perhaps. Or would it? When the health care support worker is asked for a bedpan we can expect no more of her than that:

1. she brings it to the person who asked for it
2. she ensures privacy
3. she both places and removes it carefully
4. she discards the contents appropriately, having measured them as necessary.

And this ritual, if we have trained her well, will be performed every time the task is requested of her, no matter that on one occasion it concerns a woman in the antenatal ward, on another a patient in the coronary care unit, and on a third a patient in a general ward suffering from congestive cardiac failure. The point of National Vocational Qualifications is, after all, that the skills are common to workers throughout an occupational domain and are thus directly transferable.

The casual observer will have no problem with this, as the qualified nurse would appear to be doing exactly the same. The point, however, is that she is not. The request for a bedpan by a woman in the antenatal ward alerts the midwife to consider whether the woman's cervix is fully dilated and she is thus likely to get more in the bedpan than she had bargained for. The coronary care unit patient's request could be the result of increased vagal activity and might indicate a further infarct. The patient with congestive cardiac failure might be producing inadequate amounts of urine in relation to her diuretic treatment, even though the amount could appear quite normal to the inexperienced eye.

The professional nurse, it can be seen, requires skills of conceptualisation and analysis. Where the support worker concerns herself with function the professional nurse includes purpose. And purpose suggests understanding and judgement—the very expectations that can be found, for example, in reports on the activities of health visitors in response to inquiries into deaths from child abuse ranging from Maria Colwell in 1973 to Kimberley Carlile in 1986 (Blom-Cooper 1987).

The practice of nursing involves more than that which can be seen. It might well also involve activities which are observable, but these might be the skills which are most easily learned. How is nursing (by which I mean all of nursing) learned? Are the observable skills of nursing learned more easily than the unobservable? Are they learned separately from the skills of understanding and judgement or does one piece of learning stem from the other?

REPORT ON A RESEARCH ACTIVITY

I wish to make a short digression at this point, to describe a conversation with a group of nurses, which took place as part of a research project. The activity involved a group of 20 qualified nurses, all of whom were students on a short course on teaching and assessment in clinical practice. It was the second day of the course. The conversation followed a discussion of professional issues, such as the Regional Health Authority's education strategy, a proposed college amalgamation, The United Kingdom Central Council's Post Registration Education and Practice Project, and the English National Board Higher Awards framework.

The group was informed that the research involved an investigation into the nature of nursing knowledge, particularly that

FORMALISING NURSING KNOWLEDGE 37

which is created through professional practice. They were told that a situation would be described to them, following which their comments would be invited. The description was as follows:

The ward clerk was busy at her desk, but none the less overheard the following conversation between student nurse A and staff nurse B:

Student nurse A: 'Poor Mr Jones is not going to get better, is he staff nurse?'
Staff nurse B: 'I don't think so, no.'
Student nurse A: 'He seems very close to his daughter, too, doesn't he? It would be awful if he died without her, wouldn't it? I mean, it would seem really unfair.'
Staff nurse B: 'Yes it would, but that is often the way things happen.'
Student nurse A: 'I hope I'm not here when it happens. Well, you know what I mean, I'd hate to have to phone the daughter to tell her that her father had died without her being present. It would be such a shock to her.'
Staff nurse B: 'But it isn't necessary to handle it like that. You can just 'phone to say that he had taken a turn for the worse and should come as quickly as possible.'

The ward clerk felt disturbed by what she had heard and discussed it with another ward clerk. 'What do you think of that?' she asked her friend. 'Oh they often do that,' replied the friend, 'rather than upset the relatives.'

At this point the group was asked for a general impression of what had been said.

'Quite horrific', said one.

'Does anyone wish to challenge that comment?' they were asked. No-one did. They were asked again whether anyone had sympathy with the approach taken by the staff nurse. Again, no-one did.

'Why do you think that the staff nurse behaved like that then?'

'Custom and practice', answered one.

'Custom and practice to lie?'

'I'm sure it was well meaning', she answered. 'The staff nurse would probably have thought she was being kind to the patient's relatives.'

'I used to think like that at one time' ventured another nurse.

'So did I', said another, and a few other heads were nodding.

'What made you change your view?'

'Talking to patients' relatives after the event, and asking other relatives what information they would like, given such unfortunate circumstances', she replied.

'I can't bear the idea of anyone dying alone', put in another. 'And I'm not prepared to lie just because another nurse thinks I should. And anyway, I think the nurse is trying to protect herself, not the patient or his relatives. I can understand why, of course, but it's still not right.'

'So, many of you at one time held the view that telling a white lie is all right, if it is in the patient's interest. Now you don't believe it is in the

patient's or relative's interest. And you are telling me that you came to this conclusion based on your own experiences. Is that right?'
'Yes.' was the reply.
'Did any of you support this with extra reading? Did any of you think of doing so?' No-one had done any reading of ethical issues or their solutions, but one nurse had considered a course in ethical decision making, although she had not followed it through.
'Well, bearing in mind you are content with the view you now all hold, is it all right to say that all you need is time and experience and the opportunity to reflect and all will come right?'
'No', said several at once, and one man continued:
'I believe we should be given the opportunity to work these things through. I know they say that every situation is different and you have to make your mind up about everyone individually, but I don't believe it. You find with experience that instances of the same thing keep cropping up. Time and again. I only wish I could have learned how to handle some beforehand. It would have saved me a lot of heartache.'
'I think these things should be taught', said another. 'You can learn by experience but it isn't really the best way for things like these.'

Discussion

The above appears to be an example of nursing knowledge that can be learned through experience. None the less, this mode of learning—at least in this case—is declared to be undesirable by the students. What do they mean by undesirable? Did they complain because it took too long to learn in this way? Or was it because it was difficult to learn in this way? Either might be the case. What was also the case, however, was that students suggested that it was an immoral way to learn the material. Hare (1987) suggests that although regret is acceptable following a moral decision one would have preferred not to make, remorse is unacceptable. Remorse, he suggests, is felt by an individual in response to having reflected and acknowledged that the wrong decision was made. Remorse is unacceptable, therefore, because it is avoidable.

TYPES OF KNOWLEDGE

Eraut (1985) considers knowledge creation and knowledge use in professional contexts, and although he does not address nursing specifically there are parallels to be drawn regarding professional knowledge in other spheres which are useful to consider. He suggests that there are traditional assumptions about both the labelling and packaging of knowledge. This is surely true of nursing knowledge, which is frequently considered as being of only one kind and thus trivialised as a result.

Oakeshott (1962) makes a distinction between technical and practical knowledge, considering technical knowledge as that which is capable of written codification, and practical knowledge as that which can be expressed only through practice. Hamlyn's (1967) comment is that intelligent practice requires understanding, and although he distinguishes between what he calls practical learning and learning which is apparently less so, he supports the idea that the difference is one of emphasis rather than exclusivity.

Hamlyn states categorically that rote learning and simple practice 'cannot constitute anything in the way of the essence of education'. It might be that he sees no possible connection between simple practice and what can be learned from it which aids understanding, but other writers would not agree (e.g. Schon 1983, 1987, Boud et al 1985). It is also interesting to speculate how he distinguishes simple from complex. Is there no grey area between the two? Where does the simple connect with the complex? Is he right in assuming that it is a case of applying concepts to things rather than abstracting them from things?

Within Oakeshott's (1967) view of abilities as the 'sum of a number of simple skills with a specific focus' is his acknowledgement of abilities being of different kinds. It is interesting to note that, in his opinion 'the ability to understand and to explain cannot be assimilated to the ability to do or to make.' It would be more interesting still, however, had he pursued the issue and considered how the ability to understand and explain might be achieved by doing and making.

Eraut (1990) talks of codified knowledge as the sort which is found in books and journals, the sort of knowledge which is contained within an academic discipline in what might be considered to be the traditional sense. He also recognises that this type of knowledge is not always easily comprehended. Perhaps this is why it is valued so highly. But he also properly acknowledges that this type of knowledge is even more difficult to apply than it is to learn. Eraut introduces the idea of something called semi-codified process knowledge (Eraut 1990), which involves the use of codified knowledge for its creation. He suggests that, apart from being very difficult to describe, it requires planning, problem solving, decision making, evaluating and self-organisation. It is probably this label which comes closest to describing the professional nursing knowledge which is created through clinical practice. There is also the problem, of course, of whether that which we think to be knowledge is really knowledge at all. Ayer (1956) says that 'sufficient conditions for knowing something is the case are first that what one is said to know be true, secondly that one be sure of it, and thirdly that one should have the right to be sure.'

CONCLUSION

In this chapter I have tried to demonstrate the importance of defining nursing knowledge. I have also tried to suggest some approaches to tackling this problem. Since the first European Summer School there has been considerable interest in the development of a shared nursing language, and this includes in the UK the Nursing Terms Scoping Project, which will explore the possibility of adapting the Read Code approach to nursing (NHSCCC 1992). However, it has to be said that there remains a great deal more work to do regarding the nature of nursing knowledge.

REFERENCES

Ayer A J 1956 The problem of knowledge. Penguin Books, Harmondsworth
Blom-Cooper L 1987 A child in mind. The London Borough of Greenwich
Boud D, Keogh R, Walker D 1985 (eds) Reflection: turning experience into learning. Kogan Page, London
Eraut M 1985 Knowledge creation and knowledge use in professional contexts. Studies in Higher Education, vol 10 (2)
Hamlyn D W The concept of education. Routledge & Kegan Paul, London
Hare R M 1981 Moral thinking. Oxford University Press, Oxford
NHS Centre for Coding and Classification 1992 Nursing Terms (Scoping) Project Workshops January 1993. NHS Management Executive, London
Oakeshott M 1967 The concept of education. Routledge & Kegan Paul, London
Schon D A 1983 The reflective practitioner: how professionals think in action. Basic Books, New York
Schon D A 1987 Educating the reflective practitioner. Jossey-Bass, London

4

Formalising nursing knowledge: translating nurses describing and thinking about their patients

A. Hyslop

Setting the scene
  Formalising nursing knowledge: definition and limits
  Why formalise nursing knowledge?
  Formalising nursing knowledge: key issues
  On practitioner knowledge
  Identification of knowledge holders
Methodological issues in formalising nursing knowledge
  Eliciting top-level descriptive knowledge
  An incremental approach: free listing of attributes
  Eliciting micro-level descriptive knowledge: the attribute values
  Results
  Formalising processing knowledge
  Process tracing—an example
  Analysing and modelling processing knowledge: findings and issues
  The use of higher cognition
  Findings
Conclusion

INTRODUCTION

After an introductory section to set the scene, the main body of this chapter will use a description of a project on the formalisation of nurses' pressure sore risk assessment knowledge to illustrate the methodological and conceptual issues involved. The main message will be that the complexities of this task multiply the deeper one tries to descend into nursing cognition, but that it is worth the effort.

SETTING THE SCENE
Formalising nursing knowledge: definition and limits

It is important to start with clear definitions. Put simply, 'nursing' can be taken to be of the clinical variety, 'knowledge' refers to the cognitive skills of practitioners, and although 'formalisation' is probably not a good term it can be said to mean the translation and transfer of this knowledge to a different form. The current endeavour in nursing most pertinent to this is the work to establish a uniform nursing language. And, as McCormick (1991a, 1991b) points out, this is different from that other current endeavour, minimum data set (MDS) construction. The definition, however, is about deriving descriptive terms, which in turn could become a nomenclature—a systematic list of terms used to identify concepts but not to classify them. An agreed nomenclature could be a useful product of formalising nursing knowledge, just as a nursing MDS would be a useful abstraction from that nomenclature.

A superficial view of a consensual descriptive language would be that it is so much jargon. This view would be to miss the crucial point of the exercise. Jargon, after all, can be a useful shorthand which can be transmitted economically among people who share understanding. The key point is the shared understanding. Good jargon is precise and doesn't overlap, so what is taking place between these understanders of jargon is the use of the same mental model. If one nurse tells another her patient 'is cachexic', each will understand the many concepts and implications of this statement. The issue, however, is how to go about translating these interrelated concepts and implications into a valid and reliable form.

Why formalise nursing knowledge?

The above definition distinguishes between the process and product of formalising nursing knowledge. The rationale for formalisation is similarly distinguishable. If, for example, there are benefits in having nursing diagnoses and consensual language, then presumably there are benefits in deriving such systems from the best of our practitioners. The formalised knowledge itself will then be useful for a variety of professional purposes: patient records; preparing beginners; comparing outcome across settings; and so on. It has been argued in the context of nursing model development that a 'proper' profession requires a sound conceptual basis. It is arguably even more essential that a profession has a common vocabulary based on accepted strong practice. Formalisation of nursing knowledge is therefore a legitimate professional aspiration.

It is always worth looking for a cynical reason when an issue becomes fashionable. A strong contender in this case must be the computer. However, although the mutual benefit of computers and formalised nursing knowledge can be seen at the descriptive level, the advent of the 1990s seems to have coincided with the fall from grace of the 'expert systems dream'. There is little or no evidence that machines that process knowledge and make decisions like an expert have penetrated beyond the research situation. This chapter illustrates, by way of probable explanation, the complexities surrounding such a goal.

Formalising nursing knowledge: key issues

This author contends that there will be considerable benefit to the quality of formalised nursing knowledge if attention is paid to:

1. seeking to understand the area of nursing knowledge before trying to formalise it
2. being clear about the intended purpose of the formalised knowledge
3. giving serious attention to the methods used to elicit and formalise the nursing knowledge.

It will also be argued that to formalise nursing knowledge is to accept its existence in the form that it is found. Take the case of a researcher wishing to develop a set of descriptors for a particular type of patient: if the scheme is built up from everyday language used by nurses knowledgeable in this area, then this would be a good example of formalised nursing knowledge. If, on the other hand, the scheme is more a reflection of how the researcher believes such patients should be described by nurses then it may be an excellent nursing model, but it is not by this definition formalised nursing knowledge.

In order to illustrate these issues an introduction to models of expert knowledge will be offered before looking in more depth at the nature of practitioner knowledge. This will be undertaken from the perspective of cognitive psychology. The area of expert knowledge chosen, pressure sore assessment and care, gives rise to further issues which will be explored in the chapter:

- What types of nursing knowledge are there?
- What is the nature of nursing knowledge within a domain, and who are 'experts'?
- What about pressure sores? Why choose them?
- Which methods may be appropriate when seeking to elicit knowledge held by nurses about pressure sore risk assessment?

On practitioner knowledge

What types of cognitive nursing knowledge can be considered? Gotts (1984), in a rare example of an attempt to review work on establishing a typology of expert knowledge, found not only relatively few pertinent references but also relatively little coherence between parallel work. With reference to types of expert medical knowledge (where most work has been carried out), what seems to emerge from the literature are two distinctions which are preserved despite the variety of terms used by different authors. The first distinction is the contrast between descriptive (also known as domain, factual, or declarative) knowledge and processing (also known as procedural, strategic, or reasoning) knowledge. The distinction here is between the 'elements' of knowledge and the 'processes' which are used to reason with these facts, something akin to the ingredients and the instructions in a recipe. For more on this distinction, see Friedman (1981), Kolodner (1982) and Buchanan et al (1983).

The second major distinction which can be identified is between deep and surface knowledge. What is referred to here is the difference between underlying principles of the domain (deep) and the mere empirical associations between phenomena (surface). An analogy may help: turning on a television gives a picture, but the mental model of causality varies from child to repairman to physicist. Other terms are relatively uncommon. For more detail, see Hartley (1981b), Hart (1982), and Szolovits & Long (1982).

Formalising nursing knowledge seems naturally to point to an emphasis on descriptive knowledge. However, if the goal is to build a decision support system then processing knowledge becomes equally important. It follows that these two dimensions of knowledge, applied to both experts and expertise, must therefore be considered along with the goals of the exercise. Moreover, as Gammack & Young (1984) point out, the selection and application of the methods of acquiring knowledge from experts should be made with the domain taxonomy firmly in mind.

What then of pressure sore risk assessment? Why choose this aspect of nursing knowledge for study and illustration? If a view, as unjust as it was superficial, were to be taken of nursing with regard to pressure sore prevention then the impression might be one of nurses carrying out largely manual and routine tasks, a 'mindless' approach (Jones 1986).

Viewed more closely, however, at least some nurses are processing information, albeit in a fashion that may seem automatic and subconscious. Pressure sore development is a process understood to varying degrees by all nurses. Yet a score or so of factors which contribute to risk can be found in the literature (e.g. Williams 1972). Cognitive processes for combining this information can therefore be expected to be complex. In recognition of this complexity, considerable research effort has gone into the development of aids to risk judgement. Barratt (1987) reviews eight of these essentially similar scales of risk factors, each with a set of defining characteristics for categorising a patient. Such an extensive research effort could be seen as an implicit criticism of nurses' skills, but Barratt stresses that predictive aids are no substitute for skilled professional judgement.

The pressure sore is therefore a good candidate for exploring the formalisation of nursing knowledge—it has importance, ubiquity, and complexity. Nursing authority in this area, furthermore, is legitimate and complete.

Identification of knowledge holders

Locating the source of knowledge gives rise to several issues. Do you, for example, want 'common' knowledge (which may be flawed) or is it 'expert' knowledge which is of interest? Usually it is the latter, and it might be expected that given at least some coverage in the literature on types of expert knowledge there would be corresponding attention paid to the choice of expert prior to the knowledge acquisition exercise. This, however, does not seem to be the case. The principles which guide choice of expert (or experts) seem governed more by circumstances and professional politics than by reasoned strategy.

In the medical domain, similar problems arise. Wellbank (1983) advises finding an expert who is interested in the project and articulate about skills he or she possesses, but only Szolovits & Long (1982) come near to considering different types of knowledge holder when discussing the advantages and problems of recruiting university and hospital doctors, who between them might span the knowledge domain but whose professional politics may not be compatible.

In the literature on formalisation of medical knowledge the assumption is nearly always that the expert will be one person, which given the difficulties outlined above is perhaps understandable. Hartley (1981b) addresses the possibility of knowledge acquisition from several experts and explains the inconsistencies which seem to result as being partly due to some being 'experts' but others being 'practitioners'. Davis (1982) notes that the accepted wisdom of knowledge acquisition is to use a single expert—a 'knowledge Tsar'—and comments that as yet there are no good ways of dealing with inter-expert disagreement.

Gotts (1984) has suggested that the reliance on a single expert is more a reflection on the difficulties of coping with an uncertain knowledge domain than it is on the lack of ways of dealing with inter-expert inconsistencies. A counter suggestion would be that it is the problems of co-operation, defensiveness and politics which have brought about the reliance on a single expert while no serious attempt has been made to develop methods of producing 'average' expertise from a pool of experts. However, formalised knowledge must in every respect possess a high degree of validity. Any model based on a single expert cannot have the potential to achieve the external validity that a model based on the 'collected wisdom' of several experts can achieve.

In the nursing domain, the idea of an 'expert nurse' seems to have been only recently accepted within the nursing literature. The term, however, has been applied with varying degrees of stringency. For example, Broderick & Ammentorp (1979) simply deem a sample of associate degree nurses as experts, while Corcoran (1986) demands that her sample of peer-nominated experts have previous publications. Benner (1984) sought to identify examples of expertise rather than examples of expert, and these examples of expertise were then classified into one of five levels of competency.

Medicine has a tradition of shared language and patient classification, so choosing a single expert is more defensible than in nursing, which is much less developed in this respect. Nursing does not lack wisdom just because it has not yet seriously formalised its knowledge. However, Hartley's (1981a) comment about 'experts' and 'practitioners' and the manner in which nursing research has defined individuals as expert seems to suggest a third dimension to add to the descriptive/processing and surface/deep distinctions. Osiobe (1985) has made the point that knowledge can be of a formal or informal nature. Clinical nurses may therefore vary in terms of being 'wardwise' or 'bookwise'; they may have hands-on versus textbook knowledge. This third dimension, theoretical/practical, must therefore be kept in mind when identifying holders of nursing knowledge. Benner (1984) and others have underlined the importance of establishing a consensus descriptive language, implying that experts should currently be practising nurses.

Some concluding guidelines may therefore be offered prior to setting out on a project to formalise nursing knowledge:

1. Complete expertise should not be taken as being possessed by any single nurse.
2. Variation in the effect of clinical conditions points to no single nursing area as holding expertise in all nursing areas.
3. Depth of knowledge is important yet should not be demanded of knowledge holders possessing exclusively theoretical or practical skills. Ideally, nurses with balanced practical and theoretical skills should be sought.
4. At all times there should be procedures devised and applied which will seek to establish consensus expertise and identify those individuals who deviate from the consensus.

With these points in mind, the discussion can move to a report on the design and implementation of the methodological steps used to elicit the descriptive knowledge base for the formalisation of nurses' pressure sore risk assessment knowledge.

METHODOLOGICAL ISSUES IN FORMALISING NURSING KNOWLEDGE

In this section a project to formalise pressure sore risk assessment knowledge will be used as a vehicle for discussing the issues and methods involved. The project aimed to elicit and model both descriptive and processing knowledge in order to build a computer model, which it was hoped might be useful for teaching.

Eliciting top-level descriptive knowledge

Following a widely adopted convention (e.g. Hart 1982), it is convenient to distinguish between 'attributes' and the 'values' which an attribute can take on. Hence for any given person the attribute of gender would take the value 'male' or 'female' (gradations and juxtaposition of these values are beyond the scope of this paper, indeed this author). Another term for attribute in the context of pressure sore risk is 'factor'. Hence the task in this section is to specify the range of attributes (or factors) which nurses believe should be assessed with regard to pressure sore risk.

Several methods of establishing the descriptor sets of attributes and values may be suggested. One approach might be described as top-down, involving a search of textbooks or examination of patients' nursing records. Perhaps because it seems obvious which attributes are of interest to researchers, there is not commonly much attention given to eliciting attributes from knowledge holders. Broderick & Ammentorp (1979), for example, give no details of the source of 59 attributes which they used in a simulated patient assessment exercise. Hammond (1966), on the other hand, generated 165 pain cues using the critical incident technique, a classic bottom-up method.

An incremental approach: free listing of attributes

It is possible to elicit the broad range of attributes which nurses use through the use of a free-listing task in response to a question such as 'What factors would you assess when...'. Clearly it would be of benefit if measures could be derived to indicate the degree of confidence held in the lists provided by this task. In fact there are some assumptions which could be made regarding such lists, and these assumptions could be tested. For example it could be argued from the work of Tversky & Kahneman (1974) that the attributes which appear early in such lists will be of greater significance than those which appear in later positions. Similarly, the frequency with which any given attribute is listed (i.e. the number of nurses who mention this attribute) might denote importance. Jaccard & Sheng (1984) provide a useful index of attribute importance which addresses these points.

The validity requirement was also taken into account prior to carrying out the free-listing exercise. The important issue here was to choose subjects appropriate to the theoretical–practical dimension introduced earlier. The method was straightforward: subjects were asked to list the factors which they used when assessing their patients' pressure sore risk. The listed attributes proved to be unambiguous to categorise, as exactly the same words were used by many different subjects (e.g. MOBILITY). Reliability of the classification was established by inter-rater agreement techniques.

In all, there were 566 entries falling into 23 categories of risk factor with a mean per subject of around 7 factors listed. Quantification of attribute categories was undertaken using a frequency measure (number of subjects mentioning this category) and an importance measure (after Jaccard & Sheng 1984). In this way, 12 'core' factors ranked in terms of frequency of mention and importance were established. The final list (e.g. MOBILISING, SKINTYPE) contained no surprises.

Two points can be made. First, there is significant shared meaning with respect to top-level descriptors. Second, it is not whether an attribute can affect pressure sore risk that is important but whether that factor is one which is shown to be consensually within nurses' knowledge bases, rather than within textbooks.

Eliciting micro-level descriptive knowledge: the attribute values

A patient cannot be described just as, say, SKINTYPE. To achieve a full description it is necessary to have subclassifications or 'values' of attributes such as 'type of skin B', '4.5', or even 'unknown'. The focus of this phase of the knowledge elicitation exercise, then, was to specify the values which each of the 12 target attributes can take on, so that patient descriptions are both meaningful to nurses and discriminative from other patient descriptions. The goal becomes one of specifying the microstructure of nurses' mental representations of their patients.

Although construction of nursing taxonomies of patients has been receiving increasing attention (e.g. Grobe 1991), the great weight of previous work can be described as 'scaling' exercises, with all the usual issues such as length of scale, nature or type of scale anchor points, intended purpose, reliability, discriminativeness, and so on. Nevertheless formalising nursing knowledge under the present definition is not about mathematical models (e.g. Grier 1981) or predictive aids (e.g. Norton et al 1962). Rather the requirement is for qualitative descriptions in the consensual natural language which the subject nurses use to represent their patients. Values of any given attribute will therefore be a number of word strings, no more and no less than are used by the nurses. Moreover, rather than suppose that national descriptive 'norms' exist, the implication was that the values would be local to these nurses, a point also made by Ball & Hannah (1984).

In the pressure sore project, a methodological approach was required which incorporated these various goals. The core of the approach adopted for eliciting attribute values was to use patient-focused interviews with a sufficient number of nurses. 'Sufficient' takes on twin meanings. First, along with the goal of consensus language, there should be sufficient nurses to allow shared rather than idiosyncratic language to be tapped. Second, it was necessary to sample sufficient nurses in order to represent the range of patients that may be encountered.

In essence, therefore, a nurse would be asked to give a description of one of her own patients with respect to each of the 12 attributes. This exercise would be repeated with different nurses and different patients until the point was reached when no new attribute values were emerging. A category of patient was selected according to the need to complete a spread of low- to high-risk patients. The subject was then asked to visualise such a patient if one was present in the ward currently. The interviewer then followed a sequence of asking the question 'how would you briefly describe this patient's ...(attribute)...?' and noting down the answer verbatim. Each of the 12 attributes were treated in this way.

Results

The 34 patient-focused interviews yielded data which were analysed in order that maximum standardisation and consensus was achieved. An example for MOBILISING was 'bed or chairfast with short assisted walks only'. A questionnaire was then designed to assemble a large cohort of patients ($n=154$) who were described in terms of the 12 attributes and values and who had been evaluated in terms of risk of developing sores by the nurses who were caring for them.

Achieving the goals was difficult. More recent work by Grobe and others (e.g. Grobe 1991) seems to offer methodological refinements as well useful thesaurus-like software. In medicine, the projects surrounding the Unified Medical Language System (e.g. Lindberg & Humphreys 1990) and the Read Clinical Classification scheme (Read 1990) show that mapping synonyms within overall categories is conceptually and computationally possible. Using coded nursing descriptors within computers serves to raise additional issues such as the need to define the properties such data can take on, which returns the discussion to the useful work being undertaken to construct consensual nursing language and minimum data sets (see Werley & Lang 1988).

Formalising processing knowledge

The story thus far is of assembling the descriptive level knowledge used by nurses during the cognitive operation of assessing a patient's risk of developing pressure sores. To the extent that this knowledge is valid, it can be taken as corresponding to the symbols which are used by the nurse mentally to represent the patient she is assessing. The aim of this knowledge formalisation project, however, was also to emulate the active processing of these symbols by expert nurses. The medium for achieving this cognitive model was to be the computer. It was therefore important to ensure that there was both descriptive and processing knowledge of sufficient detail for it to be encoded into a computer.

This point about the chosen medium is important. If the medium had been the blackboard then boxes could have been drawn to represent the resultant cognitive model. The computer, however, requires precisely specified instruction code. Although this in turn helps to add a certain measure of rigour to the theoretical basis of the model, the practical consequence is that the methodology used must be adequate to the task of preparing this code. This imperative, and the imperatives of reliability and validity, must at all times be considered when choosing a suitable method for achieving the more difficult goal of eliciting the processing knowledge. Three qualitative approaches or methods of analysing processing knowledge can be considered: phenomenological, verbal protocol analysis, and process tracing.

The phenomenological perspective has, as Tanner (1988) points out, multiple perspectives but also some common assumptions. With regard to the study of information processing, however, it quickly becomes clear that the present project does not share all of these assumptions. One point, put strongly by Benner (1984), is the belief that formal specification of clinical judgement cannot be achieved if removed from the context in which the action takes place. A more rationalist perspective would be that it does not follow that these same decision makers cannot make decisions on reduced information.

Verbal protocol analysis is possibly the main qualitative approach to have been employed both in medical and nursing decision-making research (see for example the work by Elstein et al 1978, and some recent nursing studies, e.g. Tanner 1983, Corcoran 1986, Fonteyn et al 1991). Analysis of transcripts taken from subjects who are instructed to 'think aloud' can provide data sufficiently rich to construct computer-based cognitive models (Ericsson & Simon 1983). Moreover, as Elstein et al (1983) point out, the richness of such data is educationally attractive.

Aside from the well-aired dispute about the validity of cognition which is verbalised (see Ericsson & Simon 1983 for overview), there are three problems connected with protocol analysis methodology. First, Lichtenstein (1982) has made the point that as experts' cognition becomes more automatic, the verbalisation from experts may reflect little more than the way these subjects as novices would have gone about solving the problem. Second, a point made by Patel & Groen (1986) is that this methodology becomes less applicable in verbally complex situations which depend on a rich knowledge base (in contrast to the 'toy' problems successfully studied using protocol analysis). Third, reliability and validity are jeopardised since the huge volume of data produced by the method acts to ensure that very few subjects and possibly a single patient are analysed.

Process tracing methodology seems to avoid the main criticisms made of the other methods. Moreover, it has been used to effect in studies of nursing cognition by Gordon (1980). The paradigm, which has been developed principally by Payne (1976), acknowledges the role of subjects' concurrent verbalisations while solving a task but goes considerably further in the measurement of the processing of information in pre-decisional behaviour. This is achieved mainly through a procedure which ensures that monitoring of information use by the subject can be carried out reliably. In a typical experiment (Payne 1976), an 'information board' displayed envelopes labelled with attribute names. The subjects' task was to search the information as they wished by opening envelopes and reading the attribute values contained within. Subjects were also asked to 'think out loud' while performing this task.

Payne et al (1978) argue that there are clear benefits in using a concurrent multi-method approach which incorporates both information acquisition and verbal report data. They found that ambiguities arising from one source could often be made more clear when the concurrent data from the other source were inspected. In the light of the criticisms of verbal comments given retrospectively (Nisbett & Wilson 1977) or given in response to specific questions (Ericsson & Simon 1983), Payne (1976) has shown that useful verbal protocol data can be provided by focusing more on the information search task while asking subjects to 'think aloud' regarding anything that comes to them.

Process tracing—an example

It was suggested that the project could set up a simulated patient assessment exercise, during which data would be collected from subjects as they searched the available attribute values. Simultaneously, a record could be made of 'simple' verbalisations. It was hoped that this experimental design would improve on some of the previous research using this paradigm by the use of a computer, both to present patients to subjects and covertly to record their responses; this would obviate possible effects of the presence of an experimenter. Second, it was intended to run the experiment with a greater number of both subjects and patients to be assessed. Third, there was not complete reliance on sequential information search in that patients would on occasion be presented with all information simultaneously available.

The objectives of the simulated patient assessment experiment were therefore:

1. To provide data corresponding to processing knowledge and hence complete the knowledge elicitation phase of the project.
2. To develop and apply methods which will identify subjects whose performance of the pressure sore risk assessment task can be taken as expert.
3. To carry forward this expert knowledge to a more rigorous analysis from which a cognitive model of formalised nursing knowledge could be constructed.

The computer-generated simulated patient assessment task is described here in outline only. A purpose-built program was written for an Apple Macintosh in which a sequence of 18 patients was presented to subjects in each of two conditions. These conditions were, first, the SELECT condition, when the 14 subjects used a mouse to find out information about a patient before making a decision on the risk of developing pressure sores, and second, an ALLUP condition when 12 of the factor values were presented on the screen simultaneously.

A SELECT screen is depicted in Figure 4.1 below. Adjacent to each button (□) the name of an attribute is displayed, although in this example only three attribute names are shown. The subject requires to know the values of some or all of these attributes before a decision can be made. To find a value, the subject uses the mouse to 'click' on the appropriate button, whereupon the value appears

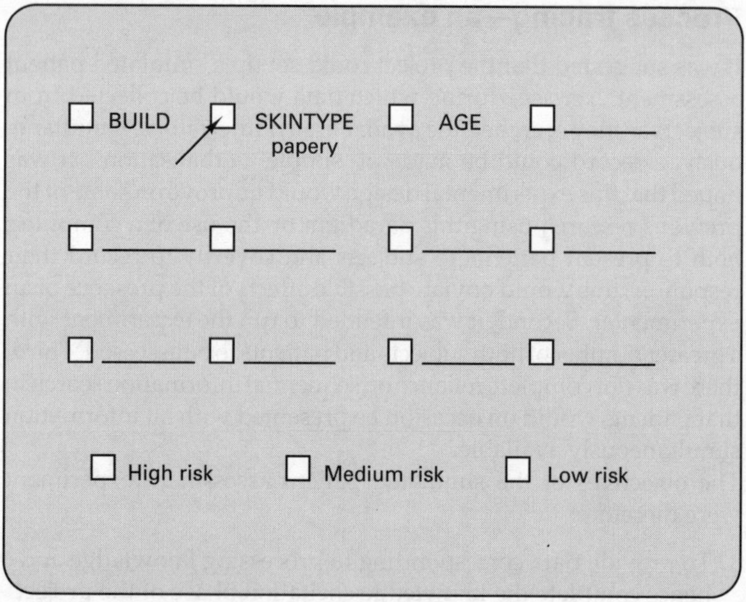

```
☐ BUILD    ☑ SKINTYPE   ☐ AGE    ☐ _____
              papery

☐ _____  ☐ _____   ☐ _____  ☐ _____

☐ _____  ☐ _____   ☐ _____  ☐ _____


  ☐ High risk   ☐ Medium risk   ☐ Low risk
```

Fig 4.1 Depiction of screen faced by experimental subjects.

below the attribute name. In the example the mouse arrow has been clicked on SKINTYPE, revealing that this patient has 'papery' skin. Three more 'decision' buttons were placed at the foot of the screen—High, Medium, and Low risk. When the nurse had elicited sufficient information to make a risk decision, she ended that patient's assessment by clicking one of these three buttons. The computer covertly recorded the order in which information was acquired and the eventual decision. Comments made throughout the task were also recorded from each nurse.

Fifteen 'potentially expert' (registered) nurses completed this task. The data collected comprised process traces corresponding to 15 x 36 patient assessment situations. The principal goal was to study in some detail the performance of subjects with demonstrable expertise, so the first set of analyses sought to identify a homogeneous expert subset of the subjects. A group of five 'experts' was identified using measures in a multivariate set-up such as decision concordance, decision consistency, and coarse indices of information search similarities. There is insufficient space to describe this in detail, but one clear and reliable finding was that more experienced nurses judged risk more accurately and did so on the basis of less information than the proficient nurses, particularly when assessing high-risk patients.

The data from these five expert nurses was then analysed. This represented a key step in achieving the aim of the project to build up and represent an increasingly fine-grained understanding of these nurses' cognitive representations and processes as a computer-based cognitive model of a nurse assessing a patient in the SELECT condition. The issues and findings which emerged from this phase are of relevance to formalising nursing knowledge, since understanding the nature of knowledge must come before formalising it.

Analysing and modelling processing knowledge: findings and issues

Once again, it emerges that the researcher must be clear about the various paradigms of nursing knowledge before attempting to formalise knowledge, this time in the form of data on knowledge processing. There are key differences in these paradigms, with potential effect on the formalised knowledge. In this particular study, the overall strategy for achieving the understanding of the experts' cognition was to keep options open by applying various 'contender' explanations to the data. Four main contender explanations, derived from the literature, relate to cue importance, use of higher cognitive processes, point for decision making, and the process of decision making. The power of each of these to explain the nurses' cognition required detailed assessment.

Reliability measures were sought throughout the project (Hyslop et al 1987). The simplest but most stringent measure was derived from matrix comparison. Each subject's process trace was formed into a 216-cell matrix (12 factors x 18 patients). In each cell of the matrix was a number corresponding to the order in which a particular factor was searched for a particular patient. If a factor was left unsearched then a zero was used. Each patient was input to the computer-based cognitive model as it underwent gradual construction, and it therefore became straightforward to measure the goodness of fit between the model's matrix and the matrix derived from each subject. The measure could then be expressed in terms of the proportion of cells perfectly matching.

The importance of attributes is a clear contender for explaining the nurses' cognition. The concept of cue importance or significance is central to all the principal theoretical models of decision making. The central idea is one of reduction of uncertainty through information gain. The interesting question, however, is not that information has differential importance but what information will reduce which uncertainty. In other words, the scheme of attribute importance will depend to a large extent on the nature of the mental representation which the problem solver is constructing of the problem. This 'representation issue', central to cognitive psychology, became increasingly central to this study of nursing cognitive expertise.

The literature in this area suggests that nurses are poor at attending to the 'right' cues in the patient and that training is required to make them better at fitting patient information to mentally represented patterns (e.g. Carnevali 1983, Thiele et al 1986, Gordon 1987, Padrick 1988, Stainton 1988). The assumption underlying these approaches to attribute importance is the hypothetico–deductive model of clinical reasoning. This model, slightly adapted from medicine (where it is beginning to be challenged), assumes that the goal of nursing patient assessment is to match top-level descriptors of patients to nationally agreed categories such as 'skin integrity, impairment of: potential' (i.e. risk of developing pressure sores). If superficial representations were optimal then it might be expected that evidence for their existence would be found in expert nurses. Nevertheless, the evidence is not strong. Broderick & Ammentorp (1979), for example, found no differences in the priority given to patient information by experts or by novice nurses. Woodtli (1988) found reasonable agreement on defining characteristics only for the key cues.

But is the assumption underlying the hypothetico–deductive model of formalising nursing knowledge a valid one? As will be outlined below, the findings of the present project repeatedly challenged a diagnostic model based on fairly superficial representation of patients.

Findings showed that cue importance certainly seems to figure in the data, as an inspection of the attributes searched at the beginning of each patient assessment reveals. The most popular for expert nurses was MOBILISING (83% of assessments) while proficient nurses, much more variable, seemed generally to prefer a combination of AGE and SEX; this is apparently a case of functional versus routinised representation. Two principal ways of ranking the factors were therefore prepared statistically—in order of statistical importance for predicting pressure sore development, and in order of importance for planning care. In addition, a random ranking scheme was prepared.

Matrix comparison and subsequent ANOVA established that only the 'care planning' scheme explained significantly more information selections than the 'chance' scheme—a finding which applied both to the expert and proficient subjects. More evidence was found relating to occasions when nurses were 'quiet', i.e. there were no verbalisations (e.g. 'so he's bedfast, in that case I had better find out about ....') indicating conscious processing. On these quiet occasions it seemed that 'automatic' processing was occurring in that it was highly likely that the next factor to be searched could be predicted by the 'care planning' rank order scheme.

This aspect of cognition can therefore be thought of as heuristic cognition—finding out the information most likely to reduce uncertainty regarding the answer. The interesting thing is that the nurses were more driven by the care implications of the patient information than by the predictive value of that information. This was one of several lines of evidence which emerged in this project suggesting that nursing assessment is crucially concerned with deeper knowledge relating to the need to deliver care to patients. The point, for formalising nursing knowledge, is that we are supposed to be formalising what is there rather than what 'should' be there.

The use of higher cognition

The central issue here becomes whether and how nurses deliberately use high-level knowledge to make sense of the incoming data, i.e. through 'deliberate' thought. In the pressure sores project, both 'expert' and 'proficient' were apparently not collecting information in a random fashion since the evidence showed some correspondence with a systematic, top-down approach based on attribute importance. Nevertheless this correspondence was not complete. Is it the case, as Nightingale (1894) put it, that 'Observation tells us the fact, reflection tells us the meaning of the fact ... observation tells us how the patient is, reflection tells us what is to be done'?

From Nightingale onward, many nursing authors have worried that nurses' cognitive activity is minimal and highly routinised.

This is seen as undesirable, hence perhaps the increasing concern to develop nursing models which emphasise a higher cognitive systematic approach. These models, often developed with beginner nurses in mind, can be seen as providing deep-level knowledge which the nurse can use mentally to represent her patients. A more worrying trend, however, is the increasing advocacy not only of more superficial representations of patients (as prototypical diagnostic types) but also of 'even higher' cognitive processes. The validity of this, it will be argued, is open to question.

The focus on the use of 'deliberate' higher cognition when assessing a patient can be seen as a 'super systematic' response to potential information chaos. Hence Gordon (1987) and Carnevali (1983) prescribe specific models of nursing cognition which go to extreme lengths to avoid the danger of nurses becoming overwhelmed by volumes of unsystematically collected patient information. The volume of information which is the proper concern of the nurse has indeed increased with the advent of theoretical models which individualise patients in terms other than those of task characteristics. Gordon (1987) goes so far as to write of the need consciously to 'chunk' cues and to organise information deliberately. The move toward deliberation has also affected the styles of cognition which are advocated. In Hammond's (1966) terms, logical and inductive inference (largely top-down) are held to be ideal while intuitive inference or the making of assumptions (largely bottom-up) is to be avoided (Lane et al 1983); however, there is now a growing movement to re-emphasise the role of intuition in nursing expertise (e.g. Benner 1984).

Hypothesis testing can be seen as the key to this trend. Early incoming information which is diagnostic is to be actively noticed by the nurse who then consciously activates hypotheses and goes on to employ maxims or rules which serve to guide subsequent search of the data in order to decide between these hypotheses. Although Gordon (1987) agrees with Benner in acknowledging that the 'deliberate' component to this process increasingly will be replaced by automatic processing as the nurse becomes more expert, there are nevertheless theoretical and empirical reasons for doubting the usefulness of this prescription for learners.

The theoretical issue requires that we look beyond the testing of hypotheses to the hypotheses themselves. Fashionably, these may be representations of patients who are prototypical of nursing diagnoses. The prototype approach to patient classification by nurses has been suggested by Abraham (1988) and by Tanner and colleagues (e.g. Westfall et al 1986). This model is similar to that put forward in medicine. For example, Rubin (1975) suggests that physicians have stored 'disease templates' of defining signs and symptoms which are activated early in the diagnostic process and tested against incoming patient data. Clusters of attributes which are highly correlated in the real world are represented as typical of the category.

However, this model contains no explicit suggestion of a deeper 'conceptual' classification of patient details in this classic hypothetico–deductive model. There seems to have been little recognition of the importance of the functional nature of the mental representation. Classification, rather than action following from classification, is taken to be the goal of patient assessment; however, nurses, it could be suggested, think in order to care.

A functional basis to representation is supported by some recent nursing literature. For example, Stainton (1988) complains that clinical judgement is not only the formulation of a diagnosis. Furthermore, she suggests that 'the meaning [of patient cues] for the nurse will be found in the way that [they] then direct CARING ...'. Although this position is not contradicted by conceptual models such as those involving activities of living (e.g. Roper et al 1985), it nevertheless sits uneasily with the NANDA model of nursing diagnosis (e.g. Kim et al 1984). This approach, owing much to the medical hypothetico–deductive model of diagnosis, can be seen as corresponding more to a shallow representation of the patient where the goal of assessment is to fit incoming information to a predetermined set of necessary and sufficient criteria. Abraham (1988) has, however, suggested a shift in theoretical formulations of nursing knowledge structures by proposing the notion of 'nursing diagnostic structure', which includes not only knowledge of prototypical diagnoses but also knowledge of the interventions which are associated with each of them.

Additional theoretical challenges, relating to unworkable demands on human cognitive capacity, will be touched on below. Nevertheless it may be helpful to mention at this point some empirical challenges to the hypothetico–deductive model. These come from some additional experiments within the pressure sore project which in essence were fairly simple, but in analysis complex and beyond the scope of this discussion. The basic design of the experiments was to give tasks to subjects which followed from a presentation of a patient in case history form. Information in the case histories could be related to either pressure sore risk or to care requirements. Three groups of subjects comprised non-nurses, beginner nurses, and expert nurses. The tasks were:

1. A self-rating exercise on how closely pairs of items from the case history were 'grouped' within memory
2. A recall task when subjects were asked to write down all items which they could remember from the case history.

Results showed good support for the hypothesis that experts actively organise their patient representations according to implications for nursing care. Non-nurses and beginners, however, were much more likely to be influenced by superficial factors such as co-occurrence of the information presented. Each experiment supported these findings.

Nursing authors seem to be firmly in the tradition of hypothesis testing of incoming data against stored prototypical patient representations, with less focus on the requirement to deliver care. There has also been a tendency to stress that this 'pattern matching' should be accomplished by conscious and deliberate processing. Certainly it is possible to 'switch' into a purely top-down processing mode, but there are significant costs in terms of demand on working memory of using this strategy (Schneider and Shiffrin 1977). Following Carnevali's (1983) prescription, the nurse retains in working memory an apparently staggering volume of patient cues, conceptual knowledge such as difficulties in daily living and functional health status, and a potentially large number of lists of features known as diagnostic hypotheses. This seems an extraordinary prescription for avoiding information overload in working memory, a point not lost on Corcoran (1986). Moreover, the cognitive processes of chunking and organisation of data are elsewhere accepted as automatic rather than deliberate (e.g. Chi et al 1981).

Leaving aside working memory limitations, the top-down prescription for assessing patients can be seen to rest on the assumptions of largely superficial representations of knowledge in large packets and predominantly backward searching when evaluating multiple hypotheses. This denotes in clinical reasoning what Pople (1973) terms abductive inference. Hammond (1966) suggested that this mode of inference represents the 'ideal' in that multiple hypotheses can be entertained simultaneously while the data field is searched for cues which discriminate between competitors. Barrow & Tamblyn (1976) provide some evidence that experienced physicians can hold three to five hypotheses simultaneously and Pople (1977) reports some success (and many problems) in building an expert system which uses abductive logic.

Nevertheless, the applicability of abductive logic to nursing is far from conclusive. Medical knowledge, of diagnostic pathology for example, is considerably more highly specified than the relatively recent nursing diagnostic concepts. Until there is some resolution of the problems which Kritek (1988) has outlined in relation to these categorisations, there can be no serious models of expert nursing based on this technique, particularly in the light of work (e.g. Benner 1984) which argues for alternative modes of inference that see a place for mechanisms whereby missing information can be assumed on the basis of experience. Induction, for example, is the process of using knowledge structures compiled from particular cases to the general case. Interestingly, Hammond (1966) actually recommends this more sober course for nurses.

In terms of the earlier discussion, a recognition that nurses assume unknown information immediately becomes attractive in that the idea fits with the principle of cognitive economy: assumptions save working memory capacity. It is significant that when the medical expert system MYCIN was reconfigured for pedagogical purposes into GUIDON (Clancy 1983) there were efforts made to incorporate implicit knowledge in the rule structure, a key point given the claim that the system was said to be a psychological model of diagnostic behaviour. A further point can be made regarding this system in that the reasoning is not solely of the backward search hypothesis testing variety. Incoming information acts to trigger smaller units of knowledge than 'diagnostic hypotheses'. The function of these rules is to direct information search. This 'forward reasoning' strategy stands in sharp contrast to the predominant nursing prescriptions, but nevertheless finds support from some recent psychological studies of medical diagnosis (Patel & Groen 1986).

The picture which is emerging, therefore, is that the ability to 'go beyond the data' is a principle of nursing cognition which deserves to be explored in relation to the pressure sore project. Two main forms of inference have been advocated. First, that information 'suggests' a hypothesis or perhaps more simply an item of information worth eliciting. Second, that information can act to permit the nurse to 'assume' a fact which is implicit in known information. One further observation which can be made is that the representation issue introduced in the section on attribute importance can be seen as central to inference in that the suggestions made above each make separate predictions about whether superficial or deeper level representations underlie nurses' mental models of patients.

Findings

In this section the analysis will shift beyond the first attribute chosen and concentrate on the tracing of subsequent information processing through the data until the point is reached when the nurse makes an assessment decision. The focus, therefore, is on the process of assessing rather than assessment. Put simply, attention is being paid to the points at which the nurse might be saying 'Where do I go from here if I am to achieve the goal of judging this patient's risk of developing pressure sores?' The position which has been established thus far is that a single scheme of attribute importance can explain the data only up to a point. Three issues regarding higher cognition can be used as a framework to undertake the required further exploration. These issues relate to the goal-directed nature of cognition, the assumption of unknown information, and the use of hypothesis testing.

What emerged from the analyses was strong evidence that information processing was indeed contingent and goal directed. Nurses did not gather information in a random fashion and were often highly influenced by preceding factor values when selecting the next factor. An example of this relates to the observed difference in the experts when they had found out that the current patient was either:

A. 'bedfast and virtually immobile in bed' or
B. 'bedfast but can move freely in bed'.

The next attribute searched for patient A was overwhelmingly MENTAL STATE, while for patient B, URINARY CONTINENCE was preferred. The difference lies in the inferences which can be made. Patient A suggests possible unconsciousness; patient B suggests that if there is wetness then there will be friction and consequent risk to skin. This type of switching between information driven and top-down processing turned out to be a significant feature of expert cognition.

Use of stored knowledge in the form of another type of inference was also observed: the values of known attributes were used to assume the values of unknown factors. For example, the expert nurses nearly always found out a patient's URINARY CONTINENCE value. But when it had already been established that the patient was unconscious, then nurses could leave URINARY CONTINENCE unsearched since they assumed that a catheter would be present. Given working memory capacity limitations, this feature of expert cognition can be thought of as representing the principle of cognitive economy.

More finely detailed analyses were undertaken of these forms of higher cognition so that some 19 'units of inference' could be established in the form of IF...THEN condition/action pairs. When these units were added to the cognitive model, which was based on attribute importance, the matrix comparison scores with the subjects showed highly significant increases. The cognitive model was now able to achieve as high as a 61% exact match with one expert subject's order of information search. Moreover, clear differences were now beginning to emerge between the cognition of expert versus proficient subjects.

The point for decision making, the third contender explanation, continues the theme of retaining an open mind when trying to unravel and formalise nursing knowledge. Reference here is principally to the finding that the nurses left unsearched much of the available information when they made their final decision, although some unknown values may have been assumed. How was it that experts asked fewer questions yet achieved greater accuracy? The findings from the previous section on inference suggest that nurses may 'know' about more attributes than they have directly searched. Nevertheless, there remains a large discrepancy between the number of attributes searched by the model when compared to either the 'expert' or the 'proficient' group. It becomes necessary, therefore, to explore the conditions which describe the point at which the information gained is taken as sufficient. It becomes necessary, moreover, to explore what 'sufficient' might mean.

In the nursing literature the nature of nurses' patient representations continues to be defined as one which involves fairly superficial knowledge such as patient characteristics, rather than deeper conceptual knowledge. Nursing theoreticians adopt this idea by stating that a decision will only be made when the nurse feels that diagnostic cues of patient characteristics have been collected (e.g. Carnevali 1983). And yet, as Baumann & Bourbonnais (1982) show in their study of rapid but complex decision making by critical care nurses, it is possible for nurses to make accurate decisions on the basis of very little data. Moreover, these decisions relate not just to diagnosis but to the 'next step' of patient care management.

A literature review suggested two principal contender explanations, either of which might best explain the points at which subjects stopped gathering information. The first is that subjects hold deep-level knowledge in the form of a biological model of pressure sore aetiology. The point at which a subject will stop information collection will be predicted by the point at which the patient can be 'fitted' to this model and when no further successor attributes are in working memory. The second explanation is based more on superficial representation of patient features, the prediction being that working memory capacity limitations will act to stop information collection when there are no successor attributes and when a capacity limit has been reached.

Testing the conceptual schema hypothesis as an explanation of the data was achieved through the prediction that the decision point will be reached when the patient can be fitted to the model with no uncertainty remaining. Put simply, pressure sore development is a function of the intensity and duration of pressure and the tolerance of the tissues to withstand this pressure. There are therefore four principal 'dimensions' of risk: mobility; capacity of the patient to relieve pressure or perceive pain; extrinsic factors acting on the skin; and intrinsic susceptibility. From study of the experts' process traces, it was established that the necessary and sufficient condition was for one factor only to be searched within each dimension. The computer code of the cognitive model was therefore updated to include this rule. Hence the factor search process of the model would now self-limit unless a further factor was suggested.

To test the second explanation (memory capacity limitations), two other versions were prepared which relied on memory capacity to halt the information search. In brief, results of comparison between these three models' matrices and those of the nurses showed clear superiority for the cognitive model which embodied the conceptual schema. Moreover, the fit of the cognitive model to the experts' cognition was now clearly superior to the fit to proficient subjects' cognition. The difference is most easily illustrated by looking at the coarse measure of number of factors searched. When assessing the 18 patients, the experts searched on average 4.3 factors while the proficient group searched on average 6.3. The average for the computer model was 4.33.

With the addition of the 'stop' component, the information search phase of the cognitive model is complete. Before moving on to an outline of the process of decision making, it is worth remembering that a separate set of analyses has demonstrated that the model more closely approximated to individual expert's cognition than did any other expert. As such, the model gives the closest approximation to a notional 'average' expert nurse. Furthermore, the model was more concordant with the experts than were two rival models prepared through discriminant function analysis and through automated rule induction.

The decision-making process was the final area of analysis within the present project. Having gathered the information, how can we formalise the way in which nurses actually decide? In a major sense, this has already been partly accomplished in that the evidence thus far points to the importance of a nurse properly carrying out the information-gathering phase of decision making. Decision making, fundamentally, is an information-processing task. Furthermore, the suggestion has been made that central to the information-processing task which this project studies is the finding that nurses are not just gathering information in order to make a risk decision, rather they are driven by the imperative of planning care. Nevertheless, assuming the expert nurse (and the computer emulation of the expert nurse) arrives at the point where a risk decision should now be made, what is the method by which that decision is to be made?

Once again, there are choices in terms of which paradigm to adopt, as each may affect the resulting formalised knowledge. The major contenders, stated here without elaboration, are:

- probability models (e.g. Hammond 1980, Grier 1976)
- cognitive processing models (e.g. Anderson 1983)
- Artificial intelligence models (e.g. Shortliffe 1976, Ozbolt et al 1985)
- knowledge-based models (e.g. Fox 1987).

Although all models were tested for goodness of fit, the pressure sore project used a knowledge-based approach. This rests on the belief that knowledge of uncertainty is held by domain experts in the form of representation of beliefs about the degree to which events are related and therefore the logical possibility and probability of conclusions. In terms of a model of nursing decision making, the argument is that reasoning is a knowledge-intensive activity which does not easily lend itself to formalisation in rules or maxims. This position fits with Benner's (1984) calls for a return to respect for the context-specific intuition of excellent nurses.

Testing the fit of these contender explanations involved formulating competing hypotheses. If the heuristic model is correct then it will be concluded that nurses used rules of thumb which are affected by problems such as anchoring. The knowledge-based approach, on the other hand, assumes that errors will be rational, i.e. given the patient information which a nurse has elicited she is making a reasonable decision. Of the 24 errors analysed, the rational explanation was found to be the most powerful. An example of a rational error is the proficient nurse who gave a 'medium-risk' judgement to a patient who was both 'bedfast and immobile in bed' and 'mildly disorientated'. This seems indefensible, but the point is that the nurse failed to elicit these problems. On the basis of the information she did elicit, her decision turned out to be quite rational. The process of decision making is therefore a vital component in the product of decision making.

From this evidence and several other separate experimental findings, it was concluded that nurses make a knowledge-based and care-implicating representation of the patient being assessed. This representation involves reference to the deep knowledge structure of the conceptual schema for pressure sore aetiology. The cognitive model was again modified to include a facility for building this representation in working memory. It was now possible to evaluate the extent to which decisions arrived at by the model concurred with those of the expert nurses. A high level of agreement was found with 16 out of 18 decisions concurring (kappa = 0.82, $P<0.001$).

CONCLUSION

We have some way to go before we can claim to have understood and formalised nursing cognitive processing. Our current position is that progress is being made at the descriptive level. Benner (1984) argues this point as the limit of what is possible. But as she has shown, expert nurses have indeed developed perfectly adequate cognition. It would therefore be useful if we could formalise an understanding of their mental representations and processing mechanisms rather than construct armchair models which may be flawed. Nursing would be well advised to concentrate on getting the precursor part right, i.e. descriptive knowledge, before embarking on processing knowledge.

One last point must to be address the obvious scepticism about what can learned from the above experiments when they have relied upon such limited information about the patients. What about how busy the ward is? What if the nurse dislikes the patient? Surely factors like these will affect how she conducts the assessment? The official response is to readily acknowledge that the situation was much reduced from reality, but that it was necessarily reduced to a point where it could be studied. Nobody criticises a physicist's model of a wave just because it is not wet; the basis of this reductionist approach is that models which take into account issues such as whether the nurse was happy will be developed if and when the basic problems have been resolved. Critics may of course suggest that the whole is inseparable from the sum of its parts.

Acknowledgements

The work reported in this chapter can be found in more detail in Hyslop (1988). As stated in that thesis, there were invaluable contributions from several colleagues, in particular Dr B T Jones.

REFERENCES

Abraham I L 1988 Issues in the application of artificially intelligent decision support technology to nursing diagnosis. In: Hannah K J, Reimer M, Mills W C, Letourneau S (eds) Clinical judgement and decision making: the future with nursing diagnosis. Proceedings of the International Nursing Conference, 1987, Calgary. Wiley, New York

Anderson J R 1983 The architecture of cognition. Harvard, Cambridge

Ball M J, Hannah K J 1984 Using computers in nursing. Reston, Virginia

Barrow H S, Tamblyn R N 1976 Guide to the development of skills in problem solving and (clinical) diagnostic reasoning. Monograph No. 1. McMaster University, Hamilton, Ontario

Baumann A, Bourbonnais F 1982 Nursing decision making in critical care areas. Journal of Advanced Nursing 7: 435–446

Benner P 1984 From novice to expert: power and excellence in nursing practice. Addison-Wesley, Palo Alto, California

Broderick M E, Ammentorp W 1979 Information structures: an analysis of nursing performance. Nursing Research 282: 106–110
Buchanan B G, Barstow D R, Bechtel R, Bennet W, Clancy W, Kulikowski C, Mitchell T, Waterman D A 1983 Constructing an expert system. In: Hayes-Roth F et al (eds) Building expert systems. Addison-Wesley Palo Alto, California
Carnevali D L 1983 Nursing care planning: diagnosis and management, 3rd edn. J B Lippincott, Philadelphia
Chi M T H, Feltovich P J, Glaser, R 1981 Categorisation and representation of physics problems by experts and novices. Cognitive Science 5: 121–152
Clancey W J 1983 The epistemology of a rule-based expert system: A framework for explanation. Artificial Intelligence 20: 215–251
Corcoran S A 1986 Task complexity and nursing expertise as factors in decision making. Nursing Research 35(2): 107–112
Davis R 1982 Expert systems: where are we? and where do we go from here? AI Magazine 3(2)
Elstein A S, Shulman L S, Sprafka S A 1978 Medical problem solving: an analysis of clinical reasoning. Harvard University Press, Cambridge
Elstein A S, Holmes M, Ravitch M M, Rovner D R, Holzman G B, Rothert M L 1983 Medical decisions in perspective: applied research in cognitive psychology. Perspectives in Biology and Medicine 26(3): 486–501
Ericsson K A, Simon H A 1983 Protocol analysis. Verbal reports as data. MIT Press, Cambridge, Massachusetts
Fonteyn M E, Grobe S J, Kuipers B J 1991 A descriptive analysis of expert critical care nurses' clinical reasoning. In: Hovenga E J S et al (eds) Nursing Informatics '91. Proceedings of the Fourth International Conference on Nursing Use of Computers and Information Science. Springer, Melbourne
Fox J 1987 Making decisions under the influence of knowledge. In: Morris J (ed) Modelling cognition. Wiley, London
Friedman P E 1981 Acquisition of procedural knowledge from domain experts. In: IJCAI-81 Proceedings, Vancouver, pp 856–861
Gammack J G, Young R M 1984 Psychological techniques for eliciting expert knowledge. In: Bramer M A 1984 (ed) Research and development in expert systems. Cambridge University Press, Cambridge
Gordon M 1980 Predictive strategies in diagnostic tasks. Nursing Research 29(1): 39–45
Gordon M 1987 Nursing diagnosis, process and application, 2nd edn. McGraw-Hill New York
Gotts N M 1984 Knowledge acquisition for medical expert systems—a review. Artificial Intelligence in Medicine Group. Publication 5, University of Sussex
Grier M R 1976 Decision making about patient care. Nursing Research 25(2): 105–110
Grier M R 1981 The need for data in making nursing decisions. In: Werley H H, Grier M R (eds) Information systems for nursing. Springer, New York
Grobe S J 1991 Nursing intervention lexicon and taxonomy: methodological aspects. In: Hovenga E J S et al (eds) Nursing Informatics '91. Proceedings of the Fourth International Conference on Nursing Use of Computers and Information Science. Springer, Melbourne
Hammond K R 1966 Clinical inference in nursing: a psychologist's viewpoint. Nursing Research 15: 27–38
Hammond K R 1980 Human judgement and decision making. Praeger, New York
Hart P E 1982 Direction for AI in the eighties. SIGART Newsletter (79)
Hartley J R 1981a An appraisal of computer assisted learning in the United Kingdom. In: Rushby N J (ed) Selected readings in computer based learning. Kogan Page, London

Hartley J R 1981b How expert should an expert system be? In: IJCAI-81 Proceedings, Vancouver

Hyslop A 1988 Modelling of expert nurses' pressure sore risk assessment skills as an expert system for in-service training. Unpublished PhD thesis, University of Glasgow

Hyslop A, Jones B T, Ritchie I 1987 The Glasgow expert systems in nursing project: from process via structure to outcome evaluation. Current Perspectives in Healthcare Computing 1987

Jaccard J, Sheng D 1984 A comparison of six methods for assessing the importance of perceived consequences in behavioural decisions: applications from attitude research. Journal of Experimental Social Psychology 20: 1–28

Jones J 1986 An investigation of the diagnostic skills of nurses on an acute medical unit relating to the identification of risk of pressure sore development in patients. Nursing Practice 1: 257–267

Kim M J, McFarland G K, McLane A M 1984 Classification of nursing diagnoses: Proceedings of the Fifth National Conference. McGraw-Hill, St Louis

Kolodner J L 1982 The role of experience in development of expertise. AAAI-82: 273–277

Kritek P B 1988 Risks and realities. In: Hannah K J, Reimer M, Mills W C, Letourneau S (eds) Clinical judgement and decision making: the future with nursing diagnosis. Proceedings of the International Nursing Conference, 1987, Calgary. Wiley, New York

Lane G H, Cronin K M, Peirce A G 1983 Flow charts—clinical decision making in nursing. Lippincott, Philadelphia

Lichtenstein S 1982 Commentary on issues in protocol analysis. In: Ungson G, Braunstein D (eds) Decision making: an interdisciplinary inquiry. Kent, Boston

Lindberg D A B, Humphreys B L 1990 The UMLS knowledge sources: tools for building better interfaces. In: Miller R A (ed) SCAMC Proceedings. IEEE Computer Society Press

McCormick K A 1991a A unified nursing language system. In: Ball M J et al (eds) Nursing informatics: where caring and technology meet. Springer, New York

McCormick K A 1991b The urgency of establishing international uniformity of data. In: Hovenga E J S et al (eds) Nursing Informatics '91. Proceedings of the Fourth International Conference on Nursing Use of Computers and Information Science. Springer, Melbourne

Nightingale F 1894 Training of nurses. In: Quain (ed) Dictionary of medicine. Longman, London

Nisbett R E, Wilson T D 1977 Telling more than we know: verbal reports on mental processes. Psychological Review 84: 231–259

Norton D, McLaren R, Exton-Smith A N 1962 An investigation of geriatric nursing problems in hospital. Churchill Livingstone, Edinburgh

Osiobe S A 1985 Sources of information in biomedical decision-making. Methods of Information in Medicine 24(4), 225–229

Ozbolt J G, Schultz S, Swain, M A, Abraham I L 1985 A proposed expert system for nursing practice. Journal of Medical Systems 9, 1/2: 57–68

Padrick K P 1988 Teaching clinical decision making. In: Hannah K J, Reimer M, Mills W C, Letourneau S (eds) Clinical judgement and decision making: the future with nursing diagnosis. Proceedings of the International Nursing Conference, 1987, Calgary. Wiley, New York

Patel V L, Groen G J 1986 Knowledge based solution strategies in medical reasoning. Cognitive Science 10: 91–116

Payne J W 1976 Task complexity and contingent processing in decision making: an information search and protocol analysis. Organisational Behaviour and Human Performance 16: 366–387

Payne J W, Braunstein M L, Carroll J S 1978 Exploring predecisional behaviour: An alternative to decision research. Organisational Behaviour and Human Performance 22: 17–44

Pople H E 1973 On the mechanisation of abductive logic. Proceedings of the Third International Joint Conference on Artificial Intelligence, pp 147–152

Pople H E 1977 The formulation of composite hypothesis in diagnostic problem solving: an exercise in synthetic reasoning. Proceedings of the Fifth International Joint Conference on Artificial Intelligence, pp 1030–1037

Read J D 1990 The Read clinical classification (Read Codes). In: O'Moore R et al (eds) Medical Informatics Europe '90. Springer, New York

Roper N, Logan W W, Tierney A J 1985 The elements of nursing, 2nd edn. Churchill Livingstone, Edinburgh

Rubin A D 1975 Hypothesis formulation and evaluation in medical diagnosis. Technical Report No. AI-TR-316. Artificial Intelligence Laboratory, MIT, Cambridge, Massachusetts

Schneider W, Shiffrin R M 1977 Controlled and automatic human information processing ll. Perceptual learning, automatic attending, and a general theory. Psychological Review 84: 127–190

Shortliffe E H 1976 Computer-based medical consultations: MYCIN. Elsevier, New York

Shortliffe E H, Buchanan B G, Feigenbaum E A 1984 Knowledge engineering for medical decision making: a review of computer based clinical decision aids. In: Clancey W J, Shortliffe E H (eds) Readings in medical artificial intelligence. Addison-Wesley, Reading, UK

Stainton M C 1988 Teaching clinical decision making. In: Hannah K J, Reimer M, Mills W C, Letourneau S (eds) Clinical judgement and decision making: the future with nursing diagnosis. Proceedings of the International Nursing Conference, 1987, Calgary. Wiley, New York

Szolovits P, Long W J 1982 The development of clinical expertise in the computer. In: Szolovits P (ed) Artificial intelligence in medicine. Westview Press, Boulder

Tanner C A 1983 Research on clinical judgement. In Holzemer W M (ed) Review of research in nursing education. Slack, New Jersey

Tanner C A 1988 Theoretical perspectives for research on clinical judgement. In: Hannah K J, Reimer M, Mills W C, Letourneau S (eds) Clinical judgement and decision making: the future with nursing diagnosis. Proceedings of the International Nursing Conference, 1987, Calgary. Wiley, New York

Thiele J E, Baldwin J H, Hyde R S, Sloan B, Strandquist G A 1986 An investigation of decision theory: what are the effects of teaching cue recognition? Journal of Nursing Education 25(8): 319–324

Tversky A, Kahneman D 1974 Judgement under uncertainty: heuristics and biases. Science 185: 1124–1131

Wellbank M 1983 A review of knowledge acquisition techniques for expert systems. Martlesham Consultancy Services, British Telecom Research Laboratories

Werley H H, Lang N M 1988 The consensually derived nursing minimum data set: elements and definitions. In: Identification of the nursing minimum data set. Springer, New York

Westfall U E, Tanner C A, Putzier D J, Padrick K P 1986 Activating clinical inferences: a component of diagnostic reasoning in nursing. Research in Nursing and Health

Woodtli A 1988 Identification of nursing diagnoses and defining characteristics: two research models. Research in Nursing and Health 11(6): 399–406

5

The need for information requirements analysis and evaluation

W. King

Introduction	Objectives
Background	Organisation of information
The development of informatics	requirements
Information and decision making	Operational requirement
Information strategy	Person-centred systems
Information requirements	Conclusions
for nursing	

INTRODUCTION

The purpose of this chapter is not to conduct an analysis and evaluation of information requirements for nursing but rather to place the need for such a process into context. It will explore the growth of information and information technology within health care and demonstrate the compelling need for adequate analysis to be conducted. Without such analysis the available information will at best overwhelm nursing staff and managers by its sheer volume and in all probability fail to meet specific requirements.

BACKGROUND

Computers and information technology are relatively new concepts for the nursing profession. Computers are about 40 years old and information technology, in the sense that we understand the term today, much younger than that. Alongside this we have seen, during the last decade, enormous progress made in the field of nursing informatics. Yet information itself is nothing new to nurses: it has underpinned the development and progression of the science of nursing since its inception.

Florence Nightingale understood the value of making observations and using data to inform the decisions she made about nursing care. From an early point in her career she was an enthusiastic collector of data and compiler of statistics, and in 1859 she began campaigning for the production of uniform hospital statistics. She drew up a standard list of diseases and drafted model hospital statistical forms, and at the Statistical Congress of 1860 the principal subject for discussion was 'Miss Nightingale's Scheme for Uniform Hospital Statistics' (Woodham Smith 1950). From their very first ward experience student nurses are collecting selected data and processing it to make it meaningful. For example, data such as a measurement of body temperature will be compared with norms so that they can be used to inform decisions about care. Nurses then, are already skilled users of information.

Clearly, things have changed since Nightingale's time. Information, its collection and use are now key issues for nurses, and the introduction of resource management and computerised information systems has led to the creation of many posts for project nurses responsible for the introduction of information systems. However, in order to explore information requirements for nursing we must also understand the external pressures and influences that have contributed to the development of the discipline of nursing informatics.

THE DEVELOPMENT OF INFORMATICS

Hannah (1985) describes nursing informatics as the use of information technologies in relation to any of the functions that are within the purview of nursing and are carried out by nurses in the performance of their duties. By this definition any use of information technologies by nurses in the care of patients, the administration of health care facilities, or the educational preparation of individuals to practice the discipline could be considered under the heading of nursing informatics.

A more current definition (Leeder 1991) suggests that nursing informatics is 'the use of nursing science, computer science and information science in nursing processes for patient/client care which provides data, information and knowledge to the individual and the organisation in such a way as to change/influence society whilst protecting the individual and achieving health for all'.

According to Leeder, the goals of nursing informatics are to provide:

- access to information
- communication within health care
- quality nursing practice, management, education and research
- cost benefit effectiveness and efficiency in health care and to
- improve the health of society.

There are a number of influences that have contributed to the development of informatics in the health service. Of overwhelming significance, however, has been the development of information technology, which has created new possibilities and new resource pressures which have necessitated the harnessing of these possibilities.

Advances in information technology and the decreasing cost of hardware have the potential to make information more accessible to health care providers. At the same time, the costs of health care have continued to increase, and the raised expectations of consumers, coupled with demographic changes such as the rising number of elderly people in the population, have put increased pressure on resources.

On the eve of the creation of the National Health Service (NHS) in Great Britain, Aneurin Bevan stated his view of the future and in so doing revealed one of the basic dilemmas faced by the NHS. He said 'We never will have all we need. Expectation will always exceed capacity.... This service must always be changing, growing and improving, it must always appear inadequate' (Open University 1985).

That statement has never been more true than it is today. The drive to achieve an efficient and effective health service demands the making of difficult decisions, including decisions about what needs to be provided, who should provide it, when, with what resources and in order to meet what objectives.

In 1983 the NHS Management Enquiry Team, led by Sir Roy Griffiths, published recommendations that outlined what were up to that time possibly the most significant changes to the NHS since its inception (Department of Health and Social Security (DHSS) 1983). Particular concern had been expressed about a number of issues:

- a lack of any real, continuous evaluation of performance against criteria
- the absence of precise management objectives
- little measurement of health output
- little clinical evaluation of practices
- even less economic evaluation of practices.

But specifically, the review team said '...nor can the NHS display a ready assessment of the effectiveness with which it meets the needs and expectations of the people it serves'; one of the recommendations of the review was that 'Real output measurement, against clearly stated management objectives and budgets, should become a major concern of management at all levels'. The demand was for information which adequately described health services in terms of what is planned, what is delivered, at what cost and to what outcomes in terms of quality and effectiveness.

The following decade brought with it a series of White Papers and initiatives which sought to formalise the Griffiths recommendations. In particular, by introducing the concepts of markets within the health service and clearly separating the roles of commissioner and provider of services, the White Paper 'Working for Patients' (Department of Health (DOH) 1989) has made the NHS more accountable for the level and quality of service it delivers. This means that information must be available to specify service delivery in a meaningful way, to monitor service delivery and to account for resource use in terms of effectiveness and efficiency. Information must be available to inform decisions about the management and delivery of services.

INFORMATION AND DECISION MAKING

The main task of those who guide and manage the provision of health and nursing care is to ensure quality, contain costs and secure access for those who need it. This entails the making of choices. March (1982) states that 'Standard theories of choice view decision making as intentional, consequential action based on four things', and he lists:

1. A knowledge of alternatives. Decision makers have a set of alternatives for action. These alternatives are defined by the situation and known unambiguously.
2. A knowledge of consequences. Decision makers know the consequences of alternative actions, at least up to a probability distribution.
3. A consistent preference ordering. Decision makers have objective functions by which alternative consequences of action can be compared in terms of their subjective value.
4. A decision rule. Decision makers have rules by which to select a single alternative of action on the basis of its consequences for the preferences.

The Steering Group on Health Services Information in the UK said that:

Such choices and the decisions flowing from them are likely to be more consistent and more rational if they are taken in the light of correct and statistical information. They will also be more easily explicable to the public, to professionals and others affected by them and thus often easier to implement. The result should be the provision of a good service for as many people need it at least cost. (DHSS 1984)

The model for the use of information (Fig. 5.1) to inform decisions is therefore a simple one. An improved information base will lead to informed and improved decision making. This will lead to better use of health care resources and thus will ensure an improved service to patients.

The extent to which this model has been pursued by those who manage and provide health and nursing services can be demonstrated by the size of the industry that has grown up around medical informatics. Information is indeed now seen as a vital health service resource and this is seen clearly by the growth in nursing informatics. For example, 400 papers were submitted for the Fourth International Conference on Nursing Use of Computers

Improved information
↓
Informed, improved decision making
↓
Better use of resources
↓
Improved service to patients

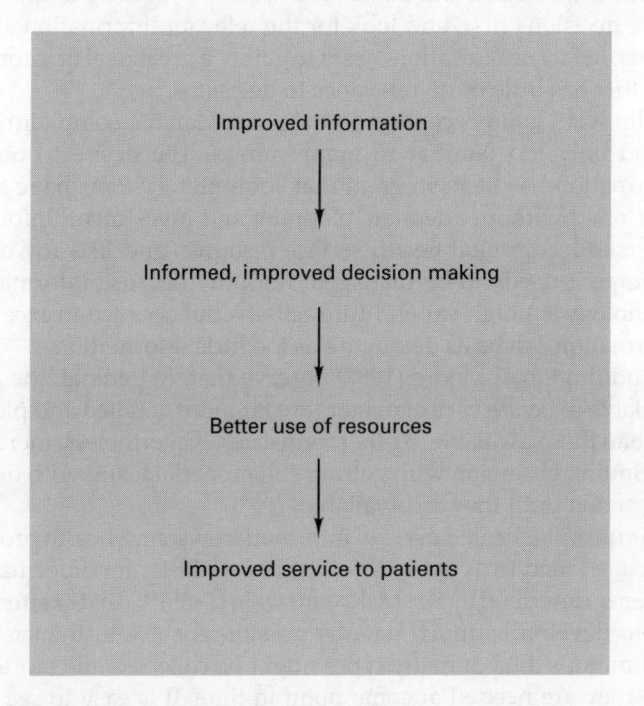

Figure 5.1 Model for the use of information.

and Information Science, held in Melbourne, Australia in April 1991. Some 700 nurses gathered from 22 countries to exchange their knowledge and experience of the use of informatics in nursing.

In the midst of so much advancement in this field, the question has to be asked: why does the basic question of information requirements continue to remain a key issue for the health service and particularly for nurses?

Having considered the importance of information to inform decision making, it is useful to return to the views of March (1982) who points out that 'Theories of choice underestimate the confusion and complexity surrounding actual decision making. Many things are happening at once: technologies are changing and are poorly understood; alliances, preferences and perceptions are changing; problems, solutions, opportunities, ideas, people and outcomes are mixed together in a way that makes their interpretation uncertain and their connections unclear.'

March goes on to argue that decision makers and organisations 'gather information and do not use it; ask for more, and ignore it; make decisions first, and look for the relevant information afterwards. In fact organisations seem to gather a great deal of information that has little or no relevance to decisions.'

The NHS is no exception to this, and March's complaint will sound only too familiar to many nurses. The desire to obtain information has been so great that computer systems have been developed without adequate planning and investment. Information is indeed a vital health service resource, and like any other resource it needs to be managed, not only because information technology is a high-expenditure activity, but because an excess of information can be as damaging as too little information.

Coddington & Moore (1987) observe that 'In general, the data available to health care managers are far more detailed and plentiful than those available in other industries. Nevertheless, there is a continuing obsession with getting still more data, and with deferring action until they are available.'

As unsophisticated users of information systems, health providers have failed to avoid a major hazard in designing information systems, described by Kast & Rosenzweig (1985): '...that of attempting to develop as much data as possible for use in the system. Voluminous data of many types might be collected and stored in case they are needed at some point in time. It is easy to see that massive amounts of useless data might result', while King (1990) has observed that 'Information mania is extremely contagious and leads units to collect every data item possible.'

It is necessary, therefore, to ensure that the opportunities provided by the introduction of information technology do not lead to abuse, in the form of the collection of data that will not be used. This is demonstrated in a discussion of the introduction of a mental health component into primary care (World Health Organization 1990):

> Routine collection of data on total populations, against the day when some specific research question may need to be addressed, is of doubtful value. Again, the problem is often one of inaccuracy of data through ignorance of the usefulness. Where a specific situation is to be investigated, or new interventions evaluated, far more reliable results are likely to be obtained by a specialised research team employing sampling techniques on a proportion of the target population.

Making sense of information and information technology is therefore a primary activity for the NHS. How can information technology and information be managed and controlled in a way that ensures that its benefits, in terms of an improved service to patients, significantly outweighs its costs?

INFORMATION STRATEGY

The first stage for any organisation has to be the development of an information strategy. This should be a long-term, directional plan which will determine what information is to be gathered and how it will flow within the organisation. This is the essence of analysing information requirements and it has two major aspects:

- the requirements of each function
- the installation and use of information technology.

Far too many information strategies within health care organisations consist only of the technical plan without a full review of what information is required to support each function within the organisation. The result, too often, is inadequate or incompatible systems providing incomplete data.

Thus an information strategy will provide a hospital or health unit with a framework within which information systems can be developed and implemented. It will provide a framework for hardware and software, secure sufficient flexibility for the future and ensure that service- or profession-specific systems will support each other within that overall framework. For example, nursing systems will take information from pathology and X-ray systems for results, but will feed into case mix systems to provide an overall picture of resource use and care within a specialty.

Developing an information strategy is a complex process. Within a hospital for example, for each major area of service provision and its related support services, service objectives and priorities must be identified, and the flows of information around the organisation must be analysed. Information requirements relating to service objectives can then be analysed, including the identification of information flows which will relate care activity to targets, outcomes and resource utilisation.

The information strategy therefore will provide the planning, monitoring and controlling medium for developing the use of information and information technology in an organisation. It is within this framework that specific nursing requirements can be considered in detail.

INFORMATION REQUIREMENTS FOR NURSING

It is outside the scope of this chapter to provide a definitive list of information requirements for nursing. This is not least because while it may be possible to agree a minimum data set, specific needs will inevitably differ between specialities and different localities of care. The information requirements for a long-stay care area for example, will differ from those of an intensive therapy unit. However, in the same way that nursing shares a common professional base and training, so too do information systems share common information structures. The requirement for nurses is to ensure that information systems provide the information structures that will meet all of their local needs. Moreover, information provided by systems should be capable of aggregation to support clinical care delivery, management of nursing resources, and strategic planning. This means that links both within the health service organisation and with outside organisations must be identified to ensure that information is complete and that it flows appropriately with the patient.

OBJECTIVES

The process of determining information requirements commences with an analysis of the business processes of the organisation. What goes on within the organisation that ensures it functions appropriately? This requires an analysis of the service objectives and information flows around the business priorities and organisation.

For example, one process necessary to support the nursing function might be to monitor the provision of service. Once this has been agreed, it is necessary to identify how this will be carried out at different levels of the organisation so that associated information can be identified. The nurse manager for example, may identify a number of sub-processes which underpin the monitoring of service provision. These are illustrated in Figure 5.2.

By identifying these sub-processes, the types and sources of information can also be identified. Information to monitor the budget for example, will derive directly from financial systems. Within acute units this is likely to present a comprehensive breakdown of staff costs, consumables and overheads. In hospitals with case mix systems, information may also be available by specialty and by diagnostic groups.

Within community settings, financial information may be less detailed and may only provide a crude breakdown of expenditure against budget in terms of pay and non-pay costs. In order to derive accurate costs of care, community systems may therefore require systems that link more closely with financial and manpower data.

Monitoring output or activity against targets will depend on the way in which targets have been set. For example, within acute units activity may be measured in terms of throughput or length of stay. Community nurses may identify target groups or programmes of care for monitoring. In this case information relating to objectives

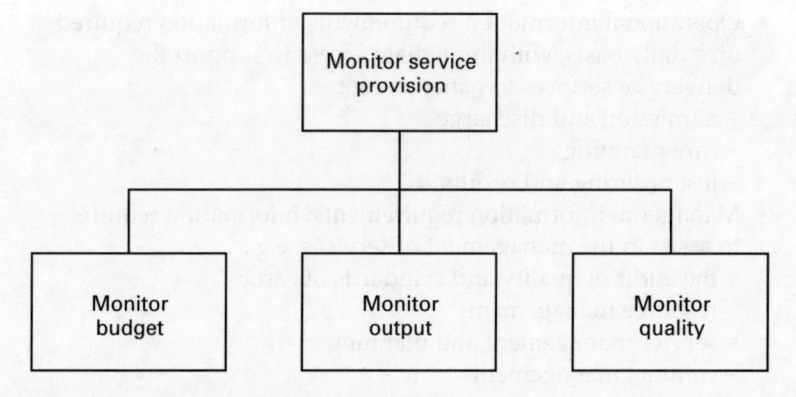

```
            ┌────────────────────┐
            │  Monitor service   │
            │     provision      │
            └────────────────────┘
                      │
      ┌───────────────┼───────────────┐
      │               │               │
┌───────────┐  ┌───────────┐  ┌───────────┐
│  Monitor  │  │  Monitor  │  │  Monitor  │
│  budget   │  │  output   │  │  quality  │
└───────────┘  └───────────┘  └───────────┘
```

Figure 5.2 Monitoring service provision.

must be collected at the time of care delivery to ensure that it is captured within systems for appropriate reporting.

Information to monitor quality will be obtained largely from the individual patient record. If patient records are fully computerised with computerised care planning available, quality standards may be built into the system for audit purposes. Actual care delivered against planned care can also be monitored by means of exception reporting. In addition, quality indicators may be derived from other information sources. Waiting times in a nurse-run clinic and patients' perceptions of service and environment are examples of such quality measures.

ORGANISATION OF INFORMATION REQUIREMENTS

Once information requirements have been identified, it is necessary to prioritise these in terms of the information that is essential, the information that is highly desirable, and information that is useful but which nurses could manage without. This is necessary not just in terms of systems design but also for reporting. Nurses and nurse managers can only use and interpret a limited amount of information within the time available to them and it is essential to ensure that reporting is prioritised. In addition, information can be available from a variety of sources including manually collected data. Where manual data is accurate, available and easily collected and reported, the benefits of computerisation may not outweigh the costs.

Information must then be organised into three main levels of use:

- Operational information requirements: information required on a daily basis, with immediate access to support the delivery of services to patients, e.g.:
  - admission and discharge
  - care planning
  - test ordering and results
- Managerial information requirements: information required to assist in the management of services, e.g.:
  - the audit of quality and standards of care
  - resource management
  - service management and planning
  - contract management
  - research

- Strategic information requirements: information required to support strategic medium to long term planning. This is particularly important in the new market environment which requires units to be much more aware of the level and type of services required and demanded by their customers.

The data collected at an operational level in the delivery of patient care may then be aggregated and processed and will provide information for the management, monitoring and planning of service delivery. An additional element is the requirement to provide information for, and to use information provided by, other organisations.

It is therefore essential to identify information flows as part of the information requirements analysis. The DOH Strategy for Nursing (DOH 1989) recognised that all practitioners will have a range of collaborative contacts. In hospital settings, for example, there is the contact and interaction between the clinical nurse and professional colleagues such as physiotherapists and dieticians, but, most significantly, in the close daily collaboration between nurse and doctor. All forms of practice represent an exercise in partnership, firstly with the patient or client in a wide variety of settings, and secondly with members of other disciplines and professions.

In community settings, collaboration will be even more extensive with a wide variety of care organisations involved such as general practitioners, social services and voluntary organisations. All of these have implications not just for information flows, but also for shared records and collaborative care planning.

OPERATIONAL REQUIREMENT

Once information requirements have been identified and analysed, they must be translated into an operational requirement for a system. The Information Management Group (DOH 1988) identifies the production of a clear and concise operational requirement as one of the key tasks in the procurement of information technology. Such a document has two key purposes:

- to assist the organisation in thinking through and formulating its needs
- conveying those requirements accurately to potential suppliers.

Compiling an operational requirement for an information system is a complex and time-consuming task. The temptation is always to purchase an off-the-shelf system, particularly when faced with a tight time scale and a skilled salesman. What too often follows is a protracted implementation period, because what is delivered is not what was promised. Systems are too often tested on site, so that months pass before they are fully operational and output reports are disappointing and inadequate. This in turn leads to considerable waste of resources, and the potential loss of credibility of, on the one hand, the system which was purchased and, on the other, the team (especially the nurse managers) who selected it.

It is therefore imperative that nurses procure a system which meets the expectations of the service and which delivers everything that is asked of it without unwarranted delays and hidden extra costs.

The core of an operational requirement will be the functional specification of the system. This is a statement of requirements which supports the aims and objectives that nurses expect the system to meet. The functional specification is then supported by a number of additional requirements including the system performance, reliability, development and support.

The operational requirement is a formal statement of what is required to meet the information needs of nurses. Moreover, it provides a document against which available systems can be judged. Additionally, by clearly identifying those requirements which are mandatory, it ensures that any system which is purchased meets minimum requirements in a comprehensive way.

PERSON-CENTRED SYSTEMS

As well as identifying information requirements for local purposes, attention must also be given to the place of information and information systems in the wider health service context. In particular, systems developed to collect information must take account of the wider NHS information strategy. Only in this way will it be possible to ensure that information flows are adequately supported and that it is the person rather than the organisation or professional group that information supports.

Many of the criticisms that have been directed at health service information systems in the past focus on their design, which may service the organisation or professional group at the expense of the patient. This leads to stand-alone systems that do not communicate and pockets of person-centred data held in isolation from each other. The benefits to individuals of a complete electronic health care record are considerable, but even within organisations, person-centred information conveys significant advantages.

King (1991) says that

> The need to ensure that the patient is the unit of analysis is a central and overriding concern. Not only would this result in information and information systems appropriate to nursing needs, it would ensure that the needs of doctors and other health care professionals could be met, while at the same time providing relevant and accurate information for managers and administrators in aggregate form. Patient centred systems would ensure that information could be analysed across time and care settings, as well as across episodes of care. Moreover, patient centred data would facilitate the process of clinical decision making, management decision making and research.

The Community Information Systems Project set up by the NHS Management Executive in 1991 is based firmly upon the concept of the person-based record. Information will only be accurate, meaningful and therefore useful if it is derived directly from clinical records. Moreover, achieving integrated health care, both within individual service settings and across primary and secondary care, is dependent upon integrated information and information systems.

This view also supports work undertaken by the Community Health Information Classification and Coding (CHIC) project (AIM.CHIC 1990) as part of the EC funded Advanced Informatics in Medicine programme. The long-term objective of the project was to produce and validate a common European basic data set which defines all the data items which are relevant to the management of health services outside the acute hospital environment and which is capable of supporting:

- linkages between related hospital and community service episodes to create an individual health career
- the validation of alternative treatment regimes based upon common diagnostic criteria
- the construction of cost models of alternative community health services processes
- the development of international standards for the analysis of epidemiological characteristics of morbidity and the implications of these for health services.

The outcome of the project is the production of proposed basic definitions of the data sets for recording contacts between health care practitioners and people and an approach to building these up, via health plans and episodes, into an individual health career.

The ability to access a complete patient health history conveys a number of advantages to both patients and health care practitioners. Patients would be spared the task of repeating the same information at each point of health care delivery, and health care practitioners would have access to a comprehensive health care summary. This would ensure that practitioners were fully informed of all relevant data about the patient such as previous illnesses and allergies, and that each practitioner was aware of the involvement of another. This would avoid duplication of service delivery, improve communication and enable a more cohesive service to be presented to the individual patient.

In order to make this concept a reality, it will be necessary to develop both the computer systems which are necessary to store and exchange the data, as well as common data definitions within the systems themselves. The National Health Service Centre for Coding and Classification is providing a coded language for health care, but practitioners must still define the information structures within which these codes will be used. Issues of security and confidentiality must also be addressed.

Within nursing, this means that there is a requirement for common structures so that nursing information can be shared across all nursing care settings. This also necessitates shared principles governing both systems development and data collection.

In a description of the purpose of the nursing record, Hoy (1989) states that the nursing record:

a. must demonstrate what care the patient is receiving so that it may be determined to be appropriate and of a satisfactory standard
b. should maintain continuity
c. should record changes in the condition or circumstances of the patient
d. should provide a permanent record for future research, teaching and legal purposes
e. is a professional document and the contents should be decided by professional judgement taking into account local circumstances

f. is the responsibility of the nurse in charge of that clinical area.

The Community Information Systems Project has also identified four principles which should govern all data collection within the health services in future:
- information needed for management purposes should be produced as a product of operational systems
- data should help staff to monitor input and clinical outcomes and to examine and improve their clinical effectiveness
- the workload imposed by data collection and analysis should not detract from patient care
- counting contacts is an inappropriate measure of service unless they are related to outcomes.

Applying these common principles to information requirements analysis and systems development will secure minimum standards without compromising local needs and demands. Common information structures, particularly for care planning, should further enhance performance and compatibility. However, the real benefits to nursing will derive from national strategies and definitions which ensure that information and information technology used to support nursing care is compatible with wider health information systems, and particularly with the person-based record. Such approaches will not compromise the unique requirements of specialist areas and localities of nursing care delivery but they will enhance the nursing care delivered by improving communication and continuity via a comprehensive presentation of person-based information.

CONCLUSIONS

Producing an information strategy and an operational requirement may seem an unnecessarily time-consuming process for those anxious to see a system installed as quickly as possible. However, as a formal way of conducting an information requirements analysis its benefits can be substantial. Only by stating clearly what is required can purchasers ensure that their needs are met. Moreover, for professions such as nursing, it ensures that their needs are understood by those with technical responsibility for information technology within the organisation. And in a world where information requirements are rarely static, it will ensure a system with sufficient flexibility to meet future changes in information requirements as these inevitably occur.

Thus the endless possibilities of information technology now and in the future ensure that only a thorough information requirements analysis will secure nurses access to accurate, timely, relevant and accessible information in a form which is both understandable and useful. Nurses and their managers are then empowered to use the information to improve their professional practice and secure even better service for patients.

REFERENCES

AIM.CHIC 1990 Community health information classification and coding. Final Report. AIM, Brussels

Coddington D C, Moore K D 1987 Market-driven strategies in health care. Jossey-Bass, London

Department of Health 1988 A guide to the preparation of an operational requirement. NHS Information Technology, Department of Health, London

Department of Health 1989 A strategy for nursing: a report of the steering committee. Department of Health, London

Department of Health and Social Security 1983 NHS management inquiry. DA(83)38, DHSS, London

Department of Health and Social Security 1984 Steering Group on Health Services Information. First Report. HMSO, London

Hannah K J 1985 Current trends in nursing informatics: implications for curriculum planning. In Hannah K J, Guillemin E J, Conklin D N (eds) Nursing uses of computers and information science. North-Holland, Amsterdam

Hoy D 1989 Computer assisted care planning systems in the United Kingdom. Scottish Home and Health Department, Edinburgh

Kast F E, Rosenzweig J E 1985 Organisation and management. McGraw-Hill, London

King W 1990 Managing resources in community health. Mercia Publications, Keele

King W 1991 Working paper four in nursing informatics '91. Proceedings of the post conference in health care information technology: implications for change. Springer, Berlin

Leeder T 1991 Working paper two in nursing informatics '91. Proceedings of the post conference in health care technology: implications for change. Springer, Berlin

March J G 1982 Theories of choice and making decisions. Social Science and Modern Society 20: 1

Open University 1985 Caring for health. U205 Book V111. The Open University Press, Milton Keynes

World Health Organization 1990 The introduction of a mental health component into primary health care. WHO, Geneva

6

Information requirement analysis and evaluation

N. Eaton

> Introduction
> **The nature and role of information**
> **Rational decision making**
>   The descriptive model of decision making
>   Prescriptive model of rational decision making
>   Rational problem solving
> **Information requirements analysis**
>   Humans as information processors
>   Human bias in data selection and use
>   Human problem-solving behaviour
> **Methods used for deciding on an organisation's information requirements**
> **Nursing information systems**
> **Key features of an information technology system**
> **Evaluation of an IT system**
> **Conclusion**

INTRODUCTION

Nurses are continually collecting data about patients to enable their care and condition to be monitored. However, much of this data remains unused or is collected in such a way as to make an accurate analysis of it impossible. There is a vast amount of data collected by the health care team caring for each individual patient, especially with the advent of technical monitoring equipment. As knowledge about medical conditions increases even greater amounts of data are produced.

The advent of technology in the form of the computer can help disentangle the data and produce meaningful information from it. Information requirement analysis is the term used to describe the process of analysing the information required by an organisation and the implementation of information systems to enable this information to be collected and utilised more effectively and efficiently.

This chapter reviews the nature and role of information, the decision-making process, how information requirement analysis is carried out, key features of an information technology (IT) system, and the evaluation of such a system.

THE NATURE AND ROLE OF INFORMATION

'Data' is usually defined as facts which are collected; they are things known, or items used as a basis for inference. They are the raw facts from which information is inferred; Avison & Fitzgerald (1988) refer to data as unstructured facts. Information comes from selecting data and presenting it in a way that is useful to the recipient, so the essential difference between data and information is one of interpretation: data are not interpreted, whereas information has meaning and use. Information could be described as desired items of knowledge which are culled from a collection of data. Information supports decisions, decisions trigger reactions, and actions affect the achievements of the information user. Information does not have a universal value; its value is related to who is using it, when it is used and in what situation (Ahituv & Neumann 1987). Burns (1991) suggests that information has become not just a description of a thing but a thing in itself and requires new approaches and capabilities to use it productively.

Information is a vital resource and needs to be managed effectively. Horton & Lewis (1991) give examples of information disasters where the mismanagement of information resulted in human misery, political misfortune and business failure. These examples include the Three Mile Island nuclear power station melt-down, where the information was generated by the computers but in such quantities that the operators were overwhelmed by it and did not believe it. Another described the destruction of a primitive culture by the introduction of steel axes when the whole structure of the tribe was based on who owned an axe. These examples show how too much or too little information can have disastrous effects on human life and well being.

The cost and value of information cannot be precisely quantified. A well known cliché has it that 'one man's data is another man's information'. Avison & Fitzgerald (1988) illustrate this point with the example of a line manager who analyses departmental figures and presents the results to the planning department. The line manager has collected his own data and interpreted it, so his results are information for him. However, the planners see these results as raw data, which they in turn will interpret and use for their own purposes. The distinction between data and information is context dependent: individuals might place different emphasis on the same piece of information, and the same information may have a different value to one individual in two different sets of circumstances (Lytle 1991).

Decisions need to be made early on about the need for information. In the NHS decisions are constantly being made about the implementation of IT. Reports such as the Korner Report (1984) on community information need and the White Paper 'Working for Patients' (DOH 1989) where information use and need are discussed, have led to computerised information systems being installed in hospitals, and computer terminals are appearing on wards. How are decisions made about these applications and how should they be made?

RATIONAL DECISION MAKING

Decisions are being taken constantly by all individuals. These may be about such things as what to wear each morning or where to take a holiday. In large organisations decisions are constantly being made about future markets, financial arrangements and the like. These decisions are based on the information available at the time—information which might later prove to be accurate or inaccurate. Psychologists have long been interested in how humans make decisions and models have been developed to describe and explain the processes. The pioneers of human decision-making models are considered to be Simon (1957) and his colleague Newell (Newell & Simon 1972).

The descriptive model of decision making

Simon's model of decision making has three stages:

1. Intelligence: the identification of the problem and data collection
2. Design: planning the alternative solutions
3. Choice: selecting a solution and evaluating its implementation.

Intelligence

Before the decision-making process is put into action the decision maker needs to be aware that a decision needs to be made. There may be two stimuli which trigger this process: problem identification or opportunity seeking. Decision making is necessary when either a problem has been identified or when opportunities are identified. Problem detection refers to the identification of anything which deviates from a plan or appears abnormal or different from an expected standard. Opportunity seeking refers to the search for other means of improving the present situation.

Whatever the stimulus for the decision-making process to be put into action, the intelligence stage requires data to be collected, classified, processed and presented in a format to allow for analysis in future stages of the process.

Design

Possible solutions are outlined, together with the set of actions necessary to carry them out. Using the data previously collected, projections are made of the possible outcomes of each of these solutions based on pre-decided criteria. The range of solutions is then evaluated, with the benefits and limitations of each being identified. If more data are required the intelligence phase is reactivated and the design stage restarted with this new information.

Choice

The final decision is made during the choice phase. The alternative solutions are evaluated and a decision made which is then put into action. New difficulties may present themselves in this phase; these difficulties might include:

- multipreference, where more than one criterion is assessed
- uncertainty, where definite outcomes are uncertain and probabilities are assigned to each solution
- conflicting interests of individuals and groups involved in the decision-making process
- control or manageability of the policy once it has been decided upon.

Team decision making is often difficult as more people need to be satisfied with the final decision.

It is possible to design systems to manage the information needed within the decision-making process; these are called management information systems (MIS). The purpose of an MIS in the intelligence stage of the decision-making process is to generate regular reports about the performance of the organisation and to provide reports answering specific queries as necessary. In most cases the information required in this stage is a by-product of normal data processing.

The MIS in the design stage should have all the data available and incorporate planning and forecasting models. However, the system cannot replace the human elements of decision making and take factors such as morale or ethics into account.

In the choice phase of decision making the MIS provides three types of information. These are reviews of the various suggested solutions, possible outcomes that could be developed as the result of the various courses of action, and the supply of feedback data for evaluation purposes.

In his early work Simon distinguished between those decisions which were easy to program for computers and those which were non-programmable. These terms later became 'structured' and 'unstructured' decision making. Structured decisions are based on clear logic and are usually quantitative. Unstructured decisions are those which contain uncertainty, intuition, trial and error approaches and involve common sense. Structured decisions tend to be made at lower levels of an organisation and unstructured higher up in middle and top management.

Computer programs cannot make unstructured decisions. They can only provide the information for the human to make the decision, such as more data, alternative scenarios, and reducing the degree of uncertainty by the use of probabilities.

Prescriptive model of rational decision making

Simon is also attributed with the prescriptive rational decision making model. This has six stages which have been outlined by Thomas (1988) as follows:

1. Define the problem, need or opportunity
2. Define what the important objectives are
3. Search for, and evaluate the various possible means of achieving these objectives
4. Select the most promising of the options evaluated
5. Implement the selected option
6. Evaluate the performance in relation to the problem defined in stage 1.

The nursing process is based on the rational decision-making model although the terminology is altered. An assessment is made of the patient's problem, goals are selected and prioritised for each problem, the plan is implemented and then evaluated in the light of the problems identified at the outset.

Thomas (1988) has doubts about the usefulness of the rational decision-making process in a large organisation such as the National Health Service (NHS). These doubts include the following:

1. Organisations adapt to change only slowly, and are rigid in the implementation of rules, which leads to conflict between constituent parts.
2. Problems are rarely well defined but rather are fragmentary.
3. People within an organisation rarely agree about the definition of a problem, or the priority of those objectives, usually due to differing perceptions of the relevant facts.
4. It is difficult to identify and evaluate the alternative strategies, especially if there are time constraints imposed.
5. Choices are always value-laden and individuals' subjective values will probably influence their choice.
6. There may be technical obstacles where, for example, information is not available or is difficult to measure.
7. There may be disagreement about how the alternative solutions' benefits and costs are weighted.

Thomas proceeds to outline a model of decision making which takes account of the theories of rationality, of 'systems' and bureaucratic politics which occur in an organisation such as the NHS, where the importance of power within the organisation is often overlooked. This model sees decisions as phenomena which emerge from within an organisation, that is, a culmination of a process where the range of possibilities is gradually narrowed as the members contribute to the decision-making process.

Psychological research into the memory skills of humans has shown that we can cope with only seven items of information (plus or minus two) at one time (Miller 1967). In many decision-making situations many more than seven items of information might need to be taken into account.

Team information processing is usually considered to be better than individual processing because it avoids the bias of one individual or the pressure of an individual in authority. It is also more successful in resolving contradictory evidence (Burns 1991).

Rational problem solving

Kepner & Tregoe (1981) describe a method of making decisions by analysing the options available (or possible solutions to a problem)

Table 6.1 Decision-making matrix (after Kepner & Tregoe 1981)

Want objective	Weight	Candidate A		Candidate B		Candidate C	
		Score	Weighted score	Score	Weighted score	Score	Weighted score
Experience as project director	10	8	80	6	60	7	70
Data processing experience	5	6	30	0	0	4	20
Will work without guidance	7	8	56	3	21	5	35
Good communicator at meetings	8	7	56	10	80	8	64
Total weighted scores			222		161		189

and coming to a decision by rational means. This is carried out by listing required factors, or wants and needs, and then assigning quantitative values to each of these wants and needs—a weighting according to the importance or desirability of each. A matrix table is drawn up with the 'wants and needs', and its corresponding weighting listed in columns. Each column then represents a different solution to the identified problem. Each solution is compared with the wants and needs and a new value assigned to how good or bad that solution is at supplying those wants and needs. A simple arithmetic calculation is then made, multiplying the weighting by the value assigned to each solution. The total score for all factors within each solution is then summed and the solution which receives the highest score is then provisionally selected (see Table 6.1).

Information is needed to make decisions using the decision-making models outlined. The next section looks in more detail at the decision to implement information systems.

INFORMATION REQUIREMENTS ANALYSIS

An information system should meet the needs of the organisation for which it is designed. Because of this it is vital that the initial stage of the development involves a complete and thorough analysis of the particular requirements for that organisation. Davis (1987) suggests that this key area is often poorly managed. Finding out what prospective users want is often difficult, and simply asking them will not always suffice. There are many reasons for this difficulty in eliciting a requirement statement, such as the difficulty humans have in explaining how they process information, the variety and complexity of information requirements, and the complex interaction between system users and analysts. As there is a variety of constraints, a number of strategies may need to be employed to facilitate a better-developed system.

Often we assume that people are adept at handling information and problem solving. However, there are various limitations to their abilities which will be discussed under three headings: humans as information processors, the human bias in the selection and use of data, and human problem-solving behaviour.

Humans as information processors

We have already seen that according to Miller (1967) humans can remember and manipulate seven (plus or minus two) pieces of information mentally at one time. This means that a human cannot mentally take into account all the factors which may need to be considered when making decisions or choices where short-term memory is being used for processing. The limitations inherent in the use of short-term memory may be reduced by the use of an external memory (e.g. a note pad) to store data being processed and by the use of technology.

Human bias in data selection and use

Humans tend to be biased in their selection and use of data. Davis (1987) and Vitalari (1981) suggest reasons for this:

- Anchoring and adjustment: Humans tend to make judgements from the anchor or base of present, known information and are slow to adjust this base.
- Concreteness: Data to be used for decisions tend to be used in the format in which it is first presented. The bias of what information is needed leads to the form the data is presented in.
- Recency: We usually remember best by primacy or recency of events. This means that the first or most recent items of data might be more heavily weighted than others which may be as relevant.
- Human statistical analysis: We are not generally good as intuitive statisticians. There is also a tendency with human information processors to mis-identify events which occur infrequently and also to attribute cause and effect incorrectly.

All the above may lead to a bias in the information which humans select to take account of in decision making. In understanding these biases we need to look at human problem-solving behaviour.

Human problem-solving behaviour

Newell & Simon (1972) coined the problem-solving terms of 'task environment' and 'problem space'. Task environment is the problem as it exists, and the problem space is how a decision maker represents the workable task. In information requirement analysis the task environment is the definition of the need for a system within an organisation, and the problem space is how this need is formulated into a model for working on the problem of information requirement.

As humans are limited in their rational thinking abilities this model is usually simplified to enable the human to manage it. This simplified problem does not necessarily correspond with the real problem. The problem space is also limited by other aspects of human problem solving such as attitude, custom, training and prejudice (Davis 1987). A somewhat simplified model of the information processes within an organisation and of information requirement is therefore used. Davis suggests that due to these constraints the information requirement statement obtained is affected by multiple factors and is only as accurate as the user and analyst can tell at any one time. Highly rated analysts take organisational and policy issues into account when formulating information requirements, low rated analysts do not.

METHODS USED FOR DECIDING ON AN ORGANISATION'S INFORMATION REQUIREMENTS

An information requirement determination methodology should be based on human limitations and should meet certain needs:

1. The method should assist the analyst to structure the problem space. Vitalari (1981) suggests that analysts spend 75% of their time on this activity.

2. It should aid an efficient search within the problem space—requirements which may be missed due to anchoring and adjustment and short-term memory limitations of human information processors.
3. It should help to overcome biasing factors such as recency, concreteness, and small samples.
4. It should provide assurance that the requirements are complete and correct.

Methods differ in the amount of structure which they offer; some have comprehensive details such as process, structure and documentation stated, others provide structure but little process or documentation. The different methods may be selected by analysts according to their experience. An inexperienced analyst may chose a method which is very structured, with process and documentation detailed. Conversely an experienced and expert analyst may use a fairly unstructured methodology, as he may find a detailed one too restricting and frustrating.

Information requirement analysis may be looked at from two levels—that of the organisation or that of the application. Organisation level information requirements need to be carefully planned to include a definition of the overall structure and architecture of the system. This plan should contain a complete set of the applications to be used and boundaries for those applications so that they supply all the needs. The interfaces between applications need to be established and the plan organised in specific sequence of events to allow for the needs of applications and management priorities. In other words all aspects of the plan are itemised in detail and sequence, in agreement with the organisation.

At the software applications level the factors in the organisation information plan are divided into subsystems which can be individually scheduled for development. Each application system is designed to process information about one activity, its design and implementation; how these applications interface with each other is detailed in the master plan.

The technical requirements of an information system will be stated in terms of outputs, inputs, stored data and processes, and the structure and format of that data. However, there are social as well as technical considerations in information system application requirements. The social or behavioural requirements are things such as job design and work organisation design objectives, assumptions about individual roles and responsibilities, and organisational policies to take into account.

NURSING INFORMATION SYSTEMS

Gassert (1990) describes a method of developing a model for defining nursing information system (NIS) requirements. An NIS is a computerised system which collects, stores, processes, retrieves, displays and communicates information which nurses need for managing and administering nursing care (Saba & McCormick 1986). The literature has many examples of guidelines used when selecting nursing systems but Gassert suggests that so far there is no model for identifying these requirements. She describes the development of such a model using structured analysis. It contains five elements or specific pieces of information that need to be included in the requirements document. These are:

1. Nurse users
2. Information processing
3. Nursing information systems
4. Nursing information
5. Nursing system goals.

The model was validated by 75 nurses in the USA with experience in systems planning, designing, selecting, enhancing or evaluating NISs. Gassert suggests that since nurses are now being invited to participate in the definition of information requirements they could use the model to help with this.

Having decided upon a plan for information requirement (whether using Gassert's model or not) the plan must be activated. Unfortunately many organisations wishing to implement information technology have already got some computers and software which users feel an allegiance to and are loathe to change. The next section outlines an information technology system and evaluation of such a system.

KEY FEATURES OF AN INFORMATION TECHNOLOGY SYSTEM

A computer consists of hardware (the physical pieces) and the software (the application program). The hardware usually comprises an input device, a processing unit, a memory and an output device. Computers may be linked together, either physically by wiring, or electronically, by communications links (e.g. satellites). A collection of computers, with large (usually central) storage and process capabilities is usually referred to as an IT system.

The systems used in the NHS have programs designed for specific tasks; these may be single, multiple or interacting tasks. When implementing systems for patient care, careful analysis is performed to decide on the functions of the program, how data are collected, stored, analysed and presented. The input device must enable all who will be using it to understand instructions or comments and input the data quickly and accurately. The processing should be fast and communicated to areas for storage and further analysis. Users should have feedback about data collected and must understand why data are collected and what relevance it has to them. Security of data access and protection needs to be considered and all legal advice followed (for example registration in line with the Data Protection Act 1984).

Many hours of analysis of what nurses actually do are needed before nurses' tasks can be computerised. Nurses tend to be unable to explain the decisions they make, as much of the analysis goes on intuitively. Consequently computer systems designed to reduce their paperwork often appear at first to take up more time than the manual systems they are replacing.

Many information systems fail to meet users' requirements. This may be due to many factors. The costs of an inadequate system may be higher than those for a totally failed system because they are hidden in maintenance budgets and staff time as they try to do what the system was supposed to do. Many systems have so much data put into them, or give so much information, that users cannot understand, interpret or control it (Lytle 1991).

EVALUATION OF AN IT SYSTEM

When designing or selecting an information system, evaluations are performed and comparisons of alternatives made (using a decision-making model) to reach a clear decision. Evaluation methods tend to be concentrated on two elements: the information system's attributes or characteristics; and its benefits. The first involves the system's characteristics such as timeliness, accuracy or formatting of the data. In the second the benefits expected after installation may be considered. These may include reduction in inventory levels, faster service, shorter credit periods and so on.

The evaluation method needs to be established at the beginning of the information analysis project. During the decision-making process the objectives which are identified need to be stated in such a way that the information collected can be used to evaluate these objectives. Often a time limit is built into the objective so that data can be collected and outcomes evaluated within a particular time frame.

Ahituv & Neumann (1987) suggest that the theoretical foundations for evaluating information processing technology are largely impractical. Most information systems are too big to isolate specific outcome probabilities, or identify discrete events, or develop rigid decision rules. Some attempts to evaluate information systems (as opposed to evaluating information) have been made. These include evaluating attributes or factors such as accuracy, timeliness, cost, or formatting of the data.

Another way is to evaluate the benefits of the installed system, for example, faster service, a reduction in man hours, or an increase in sales. These benefits may be tangible: that is they can be quantitatively assessed, usually with monetary values, for example, an increase in sales, or a decrease in maintenance costs. Some tangible non-monetary benefits might include shorter response times or a reduction in negative responses from customers. Intangible benefits are usually perceived at higher management levels and might include improved decision making and the widening of information bases for decision making.

CONCLUSION

Much of this chapter has concentrated on the role of information and how it is used to make decisions, especially in relation to the implementation of IT systems within the NHS. IT systems can help in decision making only if they are developed with the specific user in mind, after consultation with the users and after detailed analysis of information processes which either already exist or should exist. The health service is potentially a heavy user of IT and within the NHS care must be taken to make rational decisions about IT and its implementation. Nurses need to be computer literate to the extent of being able to analyse what they do with information and communicate those processes to information systems analysts.

REFERENCES

Ahituv N, Neumann S 1987 Decision making and the value of information. In: Galliers R (ed) 1987 Information analysis. Addison Wesley, New York

Avison D E, Fitzgerald G 1988 Information systems development: methodologies, techniques and tools. Blackwell Scientific, Oxford

Burns C 1991 Three Mile Island: the information melt-down. In: Horton F W, Lewis D (eds) 1991 Great information disasters. Aslib, London

Davis B 1987 Strategies for information requirement analysis. In: Galliers R (ed) 1987 Information analysis. Addison Wesley, New York

Department of Health 1989 Working for patients. The health service: caring for the 1990s. HMSO, London

Galliers R (ed) 1987 Information analysis. Addison Wesley, New York

Gassert C A 1990 Structured analysis: methodology for developing a model for defining nursing information system requirements. Advances in Nursing Science 13(2): 53–62.

Horton F W, Lewis D (eds) 1991 Great information disasters. Aslib, London

Kepner C H, Tregoe B B 1981 The new rational manager. John Martin

Korner Report 1984 Steering Group on Health Services Information, Six Reports to the Secretary of State (1982–1985). HMSO, London

Lytle R 1981 The PPS information system development disaster in the early 1980's. In: Horton F W, Lewis D (eds) Great information disasters. Aslib, London

Miller 1967 The psychology of communication. Basic Books, New York

Newell A, Simon H A 1972 Human problem solving. Prentice-Hall, Engleton Cliffs, New Jersey

Saba V K, McCormick K A 1986 Essentials of computers for nurses. Lippincott, Philadelphia

Simon H A (ed) 1957 Behavioural models of rational choice In: Models of man. Wiley, New York

Thomas P 1988 Decision making and the management of change in the NHS. Health Services Management. June 1988, pp 28–31

Vitalari N P 1981 An investigation of the problem solving behaviour of systems analysts. Unpublished PhD dissertation, University of Minnesota

7

Nursing information in support of clinical practice

D. Hoy

Introduction
Nursing information systems must be seen in context
  The nursing system in use
  Formal and informal
  Supporting action
Old methodologies have been automated in 'new' systems
  Automating practice
  System development
Existing methodologies have been found lacking
  Questions facing nursing
  Audit
  Care plan structure
  Audit possibilities
Technology's contribution has produced few demonstrable benefits
  What benefits?
  What might be?
  Standards
  Organisational learning
  Prototyping new structures and methodologies
Conclusion

INTRODUCTION

By the end of 1992, there were a few sites in the UK with several years experience of ward-based computer-assisted nursing information systems. The literature reporting developments on these sites to date has shown responses varying widely between the enthusiasm of those actively involved in implementation, and the cold water of those researchers who have attempted to show positive effects on patient care (Airdroos 1991).

A review of hospital-based computer-assisted care planning systems in the UK in 1989 found five in use, with no one system in use at more than a handful of sites (Hoy 1989). A review of existing and potential nurse management systems (Greenhalgh & Co 1992) listed 17 suppliers who claimed to offer care planning systems, with 14 of these giving a contact site in the UK. There are now very few areas of the UK that have no computer-assisted care planning in use, but even so, the majority of nurses still use paper for their documentation of care.

Some nurses in Scotland have almost 20 years' experience in this area: the CANIS system, for example, was first developed in Dundee in 1973. Based on this experience, a formal policy and strategy for nursing information systems was agreed with all interested parties in 1989. The key to this strategy was that such systems should support:

- care planning
- clinical audit
- staffing and rostering
- workload estimation
- patient costing.

This chapter outlines the lessons learnt from the progress of this strategy with particular reference to patient care planning within computer-assisted ward nursing information systems (WNIS). Community systems have also been introduced, but have so far focused more on collecting nursing activity data.

From the many issues that have emerged, we can usefully consider four statements:

- nursing information systems must be seen in context
- old methodologies have been automated in 'new' systems
- existing methodologies have been found lacking
- technology's contribution has produced few demonstrable benefits.

NURSING INFORMATION SYSTEMS MUST BE SEEN IN CONTEXT
The nursing system in use

The 'system in use' can be described as the people, organisational structures and processes which allow the collection, processing and use of information regarding nursing.

Put more simply, the nursing information system-in-use comprises such things as: a nurse talking to a patient; the nurse making a quick note of the result; the recording of a vital sign; a verbal or written shift handover; a nurse talking to a manager or other health care worker; or a nursing rota being entered into a computer. The common use of the

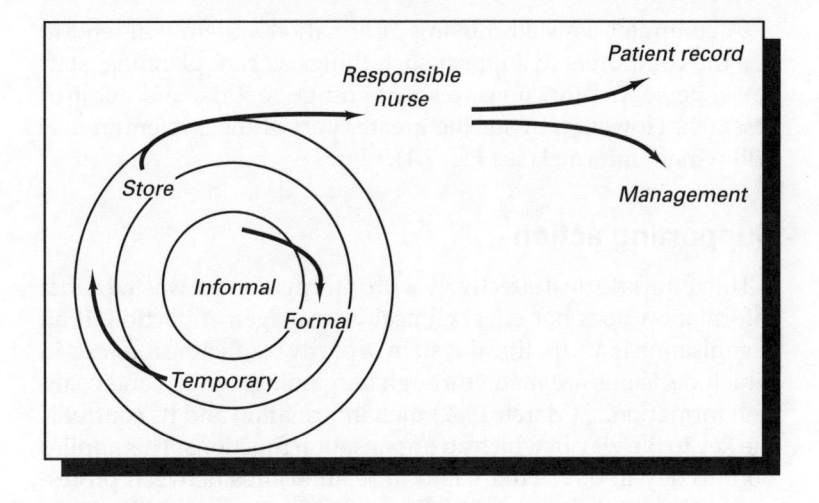

Figure 7.1 The nursing information system-in-use:
- informal to formal
- temporary use to long-term storage
- the responsible nurse 'filters' information before it goes to the patient record or management use.

term 'nursing information system' to apply to a commercial product, involving computer software, hardware and support, is grossly misleading and leads to the unrealistic expectation that buying such a product will lead to a solution to nursing's problems.

Formal and informal

An information system can be thought of as having formal and informal information systems within it.

The formal system is governed by rules, such as: a patient must have a record of care planned and delivered; nurses beginning a shift must receive a handover report; or the payroll staff must have a record of the nursing hours worked every week.

The informal system includes spontaneous, unplanned behaviour and the informal goals, assumptions and expectations that hold together organisations (Liebenau & Backhouse 1990). It is generally the case that the larger and more complex an organisation becomes, the greater the need to formalise its information system. It is also generally easier to support formal, routine information processing with a computer-based system.

A computer-assisted nursing information system will tend to use the computers to support such things as care planning, staff rotas, personnel functions, resource usage reports, and audit or research. However, by far the greater part of the 'system-in-use' will remain informal (see Fig. 7.1).

Supporting action

All our efforts to deal effectively with information are wasted if that information does not effect clinical or management action. If an organisation is a '... political system of partly conflicting interests in which decisions are made through bargaining, power, and coalition formation...' (March 1982) then information and its control is the key to the way in which an organisation functions. This applies both to day-to-day activity and to relationships between professional groups. A review of the Resource Management Initiative in England concluded that nurses had been poor at playing the 'management games' that were part of organisational change (Keen & Malby 1992). The authors emphasise the importance of nurses' use of information in dealing with organisational issues.

Interpretation of information is a pre-requisite for action. An example will illustrate the point. Suppose that a report is produced indicating that nurse staffing levels in a unit are lower than workload estimation figures suggest are necessary. A manager may interpret this in different ways. On the one hand, the report may be

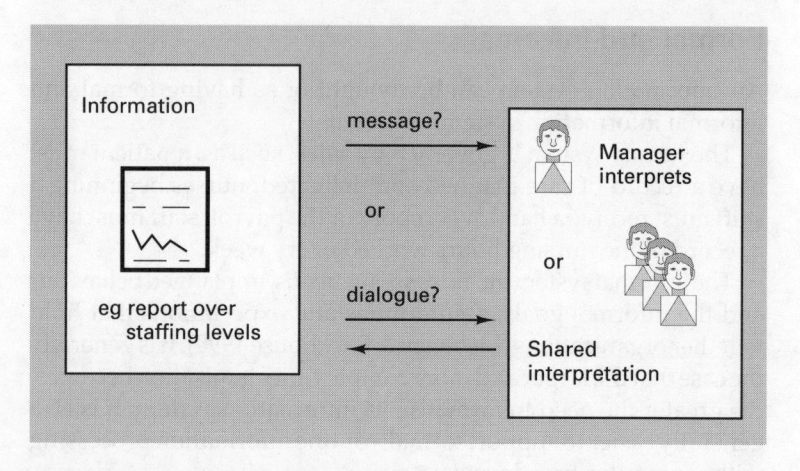

Figure 7.2 Message or dialogue?

taken to show that more effective use of nursing time is being made, money is being saved, and workload estimation figures must be unrealistically high. Agency cover could be used on occasions where there were real problems, but essentially the ward could continue to operate with the existing staff numbers. From this perspective the report is viewed favourably.

An alternative interpretation would view the report as bad news, casting doubt over standards of patient care, staff morale, and other quality issues. There might be concern about resources not used on nursing staff (funded vacancies for example) being reallocated to other, non-nursing uses.

Information such as this can be used as a message, or as a dialogue channel (see Fig. 7.2). A message implies one-way communication of a report to management. A dialogue channel implies the use of the information to support shared interpretation and joint action.

OLD METHODOLOGIES HAVE BEEN AUTOMATED IN 'NEW' SYSTEMS

Automating practice

The use of information technology in organisations can be seen to go through several phases (Edwards et al 1991). These can be summarised as shown in Table 7.1. The efficiency and effectiveness phases tend not to change the organisational form, while the integration phase will change organisational structures and relationships. These phases are not so clear-cut in practice, but it is useful to bear in mind that automation of existing practice is often a necessary phase to go through, allowing development of practice and accumulation of valuable experience. Thus, for example, we have seen the automation of care planning based on clumsy paper-based methods, and workload estimation based on methods which are poorly developed and misunderstood.

Table 7.1 Phases in the use of information technology in organisations (after Edwards et al 1991)

Efficiency	Effectiveness	Integration
Payroll	Management information systems	Standards
Accounts	Care planning	Contracting
Bed state	Resource use	Collaborative care planning

System development

This situation is unlikely to change without new techniques for system development. Traditional approaches have required the hard specification of requirements at an early stage before coding

Questions

what care?

what cost? what standards?

Answers

appropriate care

resources used expected outcomes

Information available

what was planned?
- care planned

who was to do it?
- resources required/available

what was the aim?
- patient needs

Information required

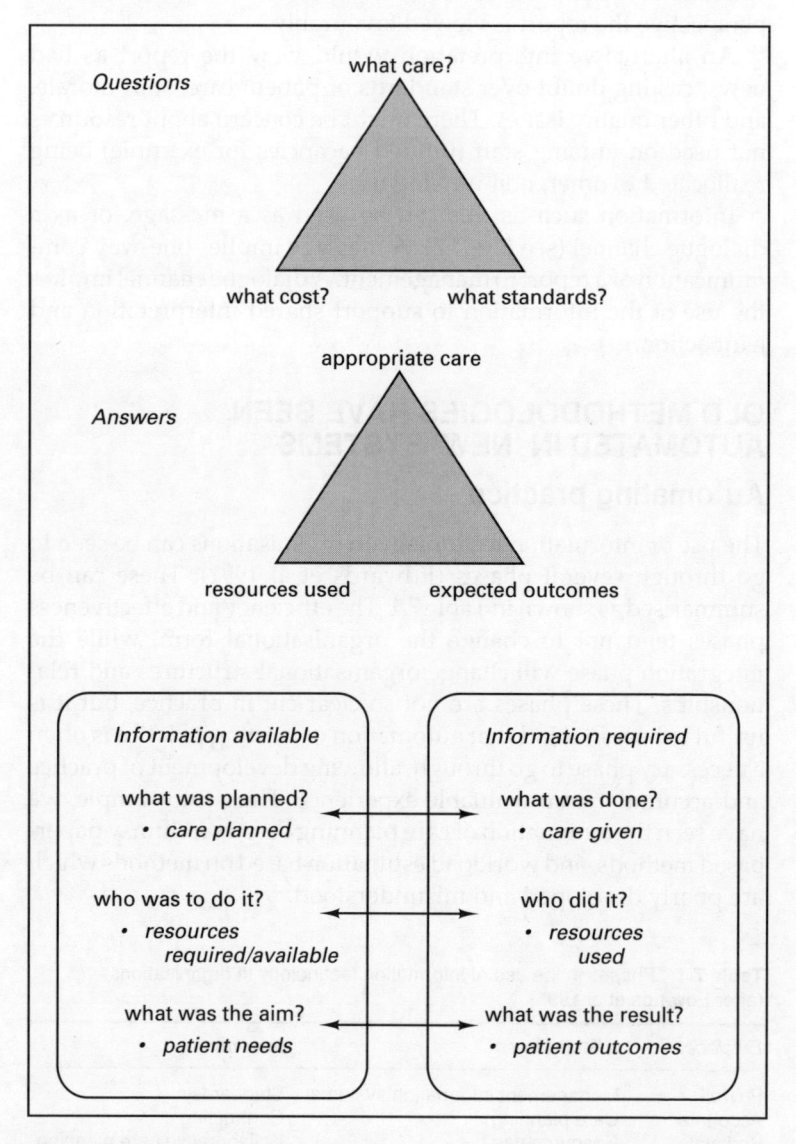

what was done?
- care given

who did it?
- resources used

what was the result?
- patient outcomes

Figure 7.3 Questions facing nursing.

takes place. By the time the user gets to use a system, it is too late to make other than minor, often cosmetic, changes. The costs of bespoke system development are generally prohibitive, meaning that 'off-the-shelf' packages are usually bought and then have to be modified to meet actual user requirements.

However, new techniques offer increasingly sophisticated development tools allowing prototyping at an early stage, and very flexible interface development. If underlying data sets are specified, then software developers are constrained to meet user requirements, and develop systems which will work on these data sets and allow sharing of data. More open systems will result.

EXISTING METHODOLOGIES HAVE BEEN FOUND LACKING
Questions facing nursing

Figure 7.3 outlines three questions facing nursing. Given any patient:

- What care is appropriate?
- To what standard is it required?
- What resources do we require to deliver it?

Given these questions, our computer-assisted nursing information systems will store a plan of care required, resources planned and available, and some evaluation of that plan. However, areas of information still lacking include: a record of what was actually done; the resources actually used; and the patient outcomes.

One issue that is particularly contentious is that of workload estimation. Current techniques are criticised as unrepresentative of what nursing is all about, or time consuming to set up and use, or simply unreliable without great effort to customise them to each practice setting.

Audit

While computer-assisted care planning is seen simply as a way of automating the production of the patient record, development will be slow and a backlash from disgruntled users can be expected in the form of growing criticism. The key to bringing about change may lie in the use of care-planning data to support audit. The use of this data to inform practice is quite new for most users, and a powerful means for changing attitudes.

By using audit as a means of exploring care-planning data we can develop current systems to their limits and maximise benefits from existing investment. Remaining inadequacies will be apparent to users, gaining commitment to change and guiding development. The audit of patient care has become an area of frenetic activity over recent years. This can be attributed to two main factors:

- the need for much tighter control over resources
- the professional aspirations of nurses.

The first factor explains the recent availability of funding to promote audit, while the second explains the readiness of nurses to exploit it.

The care planning capacities of existing computer-based systems have tended towards the speedy production of paperwork. As a result, they readily accept clinical data and produce paper plans at the touch of very few buttons. However, there is little evidence that this rich source of clinical information is easily available to meet the professional curiosity of nurse users.

The current shift towards 'open systems', with the specification of common technical standards, is bringing new opportunities to change this situation. Nursing data has previously been stored in proprietary 'closed' data structures with formats jealously guarded by suppliers. Open systems will require these data to be addressable through standard query languages. The prospect is now growing for nurses to use audit software to move beyond the standard reporting capabilities of present systems.

Care plan structure

Generally, computer-assisted care-planning systems have used current interpretations of the systematic approach (nursing process). This has resulted in a text-based record, structured hierarchically by:

- assessment heading
- diagnosis/problem/statement of need
- goal/expected outcome
- intervention/nursing action
- evaluation/actual outcome.

Some systems use internal codes to ease the storage and processing of all this text. Most allow additional free text or editing of standard terms to increase flexibility and individualisation of care plans.

Audit possibilities

This structure allows the potential for audit of patient 'type', for example by nursing diagnosis. Used with some demographic data which will record age and sex, patient movements, admission and discharge dates and types, this can provide straightforward statistics on the client group for ward nurses. Changes in this data over time could be linked with workload estimation data to illustrate patterns in nursing activity. The recording of expected outcomes with actual outcomes can allow the monitoring of standards of care: expected outcomes are based on standards, and actual outcomes allow audit of care and the standards themselves.

Experience with care planning in the UK suggests that the use of standard or 'core' care plans has developed from an early attempt to reduce the chore factor in care planning to the emergence of ad hoc standards of care. Typically, groups of ward nurses meet to consider the question 'what care is required by patients with these needs?', and a statement reflecting an acceptable standard of nursing care is born.

Figure 7.4 shows a graph based on data captured from an operational system. It shows that pain-related goals are the most frequently occurring with this group of patients. It might cause the nurses in this area to question the sizeable number of occasions

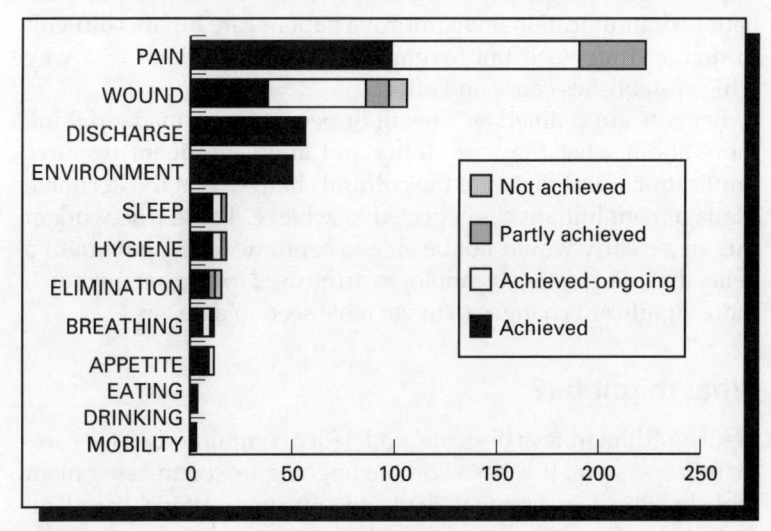

Figure 7.4 Number of final evaluations of goals grouped by assessment key words.

(25) when pain-related goals were evaluated as 'partly achieved', or the 20 occasions when wound-related goals were evaluated as 'partly' or 'not achieved'. On reflection, if a problem is suspected with care in these areas, more sensitive measures could be introduced, standard-setting done, practice changed and evaluation of effects completed.

In general, audit requires the collection and processing of additional information, for example, patient satisfaction questionnaires, or, at best, time-consuming processing of existing data, for example, data on hospital-acquired infection. The development of computer-based nursing documentation can automate much of this processing, providing the data required is already being recorded routinely, as in the example above.

TECHNOLOGY'S CONTRIBUTION HAS PRODUCED FEW DEMONSTRABLE BENEFITS
What benefits?

Expectations that computer-assisted nursing information systems would provide such benefits as savings in time and reductions in paperwork have not been confirmed by experience in the UK. Improving the legibility and completeness of care plans, with better communication, may improve patient care but it is difficult to demonstrate such improvements or to relate them in a way which establishes cause and effect.

Benefits are claimed as a result of people being made to think more about what they are doing and any consequent resource implications, and these are the cultural changes that the Resource Management Initiative is expected to achieve. Those who work in this area clearly would not be able to continue for long without a belief that information technology can be used to bring about much more significant changes than we have seen to date.

What might be?

Figure 7.5 illustrates a possible model for a computer-assisted care-planning system. It is based on the ongoing use of an assessment tool, in which assessment leads to outcome criteria based on standards of care, and which includes continuing reassessment against these standards.

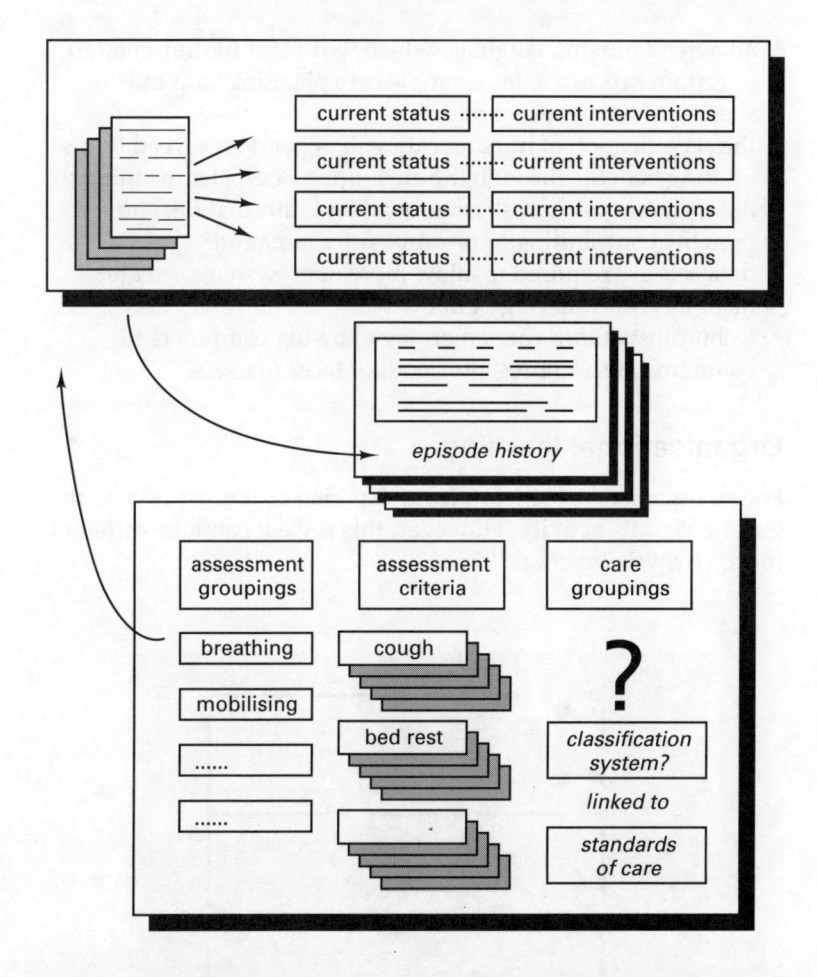

Figure 7.5 Suggested model for a nursing information system.

A classification system based on patient needs for care would support such a system.

Standards

Underpinning the development of such a model are standards covering several areas:

- agreed standards of patient care

- an agreed nursing language which will assist the automation of certain processes, for example care planning, and the sharing of the resultant data
- the classification of nursing care will depend on agreed terms, offering benefits through the attribution of greater meaning to data, greater use and sharing of patient information, and possibly contributing to resource use estimation
- data sets are required to allow more open systems, greater flexibility, and sharing of data
- technical standards are emerging allowing computers to communicate and present friendlier faces to users.

Organisational learning

For an organisation to learn from experience, it must review the outcomes of its activity. However, this review can take different forms (Argyris & Schon 1978).

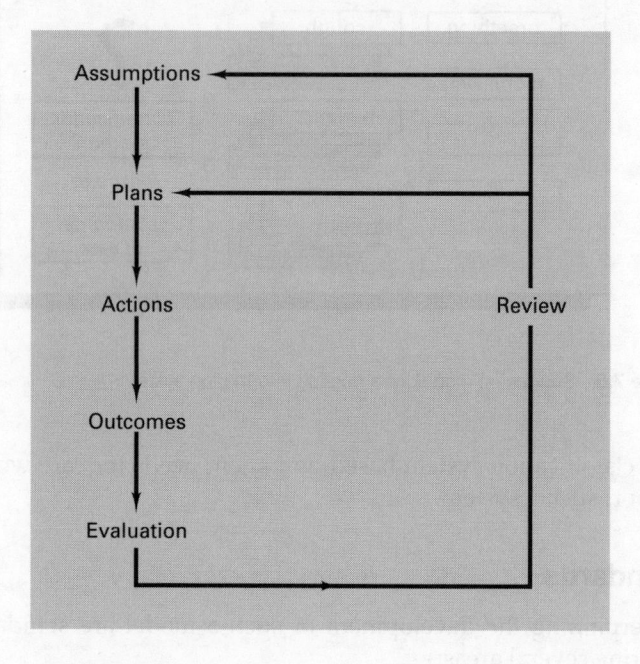

Figure 7.6 Organisational learning.

For example, outcomes can simply be compared to the original objectives and adjustments made to plans to improve future outcomes (see Fig. 7.6). For example, the review might find that a computer-assisted care-planning system was slow and awkward to use. A new improved system might be implemented as a result.

An alternative form of review would raise questions regarding the original assumptions that shaped the plans. For example, experience with a poor care-planning system might raise fundamental questions about the benefits to be obtained from systems of this type, and might thus lead to new thinking on the process of care planning itself.

This kind of learning has a more profound effect on the organisation. It relies on our abilities to think beyond our immediate situation and see possibilities for change.

Prototyping new structures and methodologies

Technology has made available new, more powerful, and more user-friendly personal computer packages able to access 'open' data over computer networks. These tools offer the flexibility and accessibility required for projects which bring together skilled users with ward nurses to allow exploration of potential in systems and data. Such small-scale prototyping projects can guide the development of methods, e.g. new forms of care planning, or multidisciplinary records. Results can be achieved more quickly, using fewer resources, and should be closer to requirements because of early user involvement.

CONCLUSION

Many of the information requirements for management and research functions hinge on the success of clinical systems in capturing patient or client-related data. Unless users perceive the effort of using these systems as worthwhile, the systems will fail.

Such high expectations of clinical systems depend on the development of effective and efficient care planning. While 'user-friendliness' is often seen as the critical success factor, good design will require that data entry be reduced to the minimum necessary.

There is scope for the simplification of care-planning methods, with more emphasis on ongoing evaluation and outcomes, while technology can automate the new processes which might result.

System design will focus on functionality rather than the professional group, so, for example, care planning may be multidisciplinary and contribute to a shared person-based record. Data regarding resource use or patient costing will require integration with the clinical record, at least to allow quality audit.

Work on classification and clinical language will depend on user involvement and professional ownership. Demonstrable benefits produced by small-scale prototyping projects will help achieve this.

Finally, in considering how an organisation (or a profession) might learn from experience, we must emphasise the importance of education. The ability of nurses to make the most of information and the technology which offers access to it, relies on a sound preparation for the clinical nurse. The basic foundation of this preparation is a clear idea of what nurses, and nursing, are trying to do with that information.

REFERENCES

Airdroos N 1991 Use and effectiveness of psychiatric nursing care plans. Journal of Advanced Nursing 16: 177–181

Argyris C, Schon D 1978 Organisational learning. Addison Wesley, Reading, Massachusetts

Edwards C, Ward J, Bytheway A 1991 The essence of information systems. Prentice-Hall, London

Greenhalgh & Co. 1992 Nurse management systems: a guide to existing and potential products. Produced for Resource Management Initiative, Department of Health, London

Hoy J D 1989 Computer assisted nursing care planning systems in the United Kingdom. Nursing Division, Scottish Home and Health Department, Edinburgh

Keen J, Malby R 1992 Nursing power and practice in the United Kingdom National Health Service. Journal of Advanced Nursing 17: 863–870

Liebenau J, Backhouse J 1990 Understanding information: an introduction. Macmillan, Basingstoke

March J G 1982 Theories of choice and making decisions. Social Science and Modern Society 20: 1

8

PAWMEX—an expert system prototype to assist pressure sore risk assessment and wound management*

N. Woolley

Introduction	Software development
Pressure sore management:	The completed knowledge base
the background	System operation
Extrinsic	System evaluation
Intrinsic	Implications for nursing
The research problem	Conclusions
Software selection	

INTRODUCTION

Nursing is rapidly realising the benefits which information technology (IT) can offer in terms of improved services for clients. Recent years have witnessed a dramatic increase in the use of nursing management and information systems. Such developments have been met by some with open arms whilst others have shown much scepticism; the integration of IT within the health care environment has not always been (and is still not) an easy task. Alongside this picture of evolution in clinical practice, nurse education is also undergoing much change in response to the predicted health care needs of the future. As the 21st century approaches, Project 2000 (UKCC 1986) heralds a new era for the preparation of the nurses who will meet this new role. IT for nursing will be an essential feature of the new curriculum.

Among other things, Project 2000 attempts to encourage the development of a 'knowledgeable doer': a practitioner armed with enhanced cognitive and analytical skills able to cope effectively with decision making and problem solving within the clinical environment. It has been suggested that the teaching strategies adopted to achieve these aims might include the use of simulation

---

*This chapter is an expanded version of a paper which received the 1991 Dame Phyllis Friend Award of the British Computer Society Nursing Specialist Group and was published in Information Technology in Nursing (Woolley 1992).

exercises (Munro 1982, de Tornyay & Thompson 1987), or experiential learning methods based around clinical visits (Burnard 1987, Merchant 1989). However, IT can also provide us with tools to facilitate the learning process and which can act as 'intelligent' advisers to the nurse clinician. These tools are expert systems.

Expert systems are computer applications capable of performing complex problem-solving or decision-making tasks within a particular area of expertise. Their design and construction involves the capture of expert knowledge, from one or more sources such as acknowledged experts in the field or from the literature, and the structuring of such knowledge according to sets of principles or rules which mimic the way in which the expert functions. When consulted, the expert system will typically seek information from the user about the specific case or problem under consideration, and will then provide solutions or make recommendations based on the knowledge and the decision rules built in to the system. Expert systems can thus function as learning aids, to allow novices to test their decision making against that of the expert, or as decision support systems to assist any practitioner in their choice of action.

This chapter briefly outlines the development of PAWMEX, an expert system prototype designed to act as both decision support tool and learning aid within the complex field of pressure sore risk assessment and wound management. The project described here was undertaken during the final year of study for the degree of Master of Nursing at the University of Wales (Woolley 1990).

PRESSURE SORE MANAGEMENT: THE BACKGROUND

The problem of pressure sores will be familiar to all nurses and will, therefore, receive only a brief mention. Pressure sores are one of the major complications of prolonged bed rest or inactivity and have been shown to have a complex aetiology involving both intrinsic and extrinsic factors. Gould (1985, 1986) suggests it is an area of nursing knowledge which is poorly understood by many nurses. The following predisposing factors are those most frequently cited in the literature:

Extrinsic
- Pressure (Norton et al 1962, Barton & Barton 1981)
- Shearing and friction (Reichel 1958, Lowthian 1979).

Intrinsic

- Age (Norton et al 1962, Ek & Boman 1982, David et al 1983)
- Moisture (Norton et al 1962, Jordan & Clark 1977, Goldstone & Goldstone 1982, Ek & Boman 1982)
- Mobility (Norton et al 1962, David et al 1983, Semple 1987, Nyquist & Hawthorn 1987, Gebhardt 1987)
- Mental status (Norton et al 1962, Gosnell 1987)
- Nutritional status (Pajk et al 1986, Holmes et al 1987, Braden & Bergstrom 1987)
- Anaemia (Vasile & Chatin 1972, Torrance 1983)
- Concurrent illness (Versluysen 1986, and many of those already cited)
- Medication, e.g. steroids (Luckman & Sorenson 1980) cytotoxics (BNF 1989).

With a view to early identification of those individuals who may be at risk of pressure sore development, a number of assessment tools have been designed, based upon these factors. Perhaps the two most widely known to nurses in this country are the Norton (Norton et al 1962) and Waterlow (Waterlow 1987) scales. These tools allow the collection of relevant information in a methodical manner and offer risk-predictive data in the form of a score for each individual patient. However, research by Jones (1986) suggests that nurses often use such tools inaccurately in a mechanistic and routinised manner, displaying little or no evidence of cognitive problem-solving skills. Inter-user reliability is often low with wide discrepancies existing between different nurses' assessments of the same patient. Given that risk assessment is essentially a problem-solving activity, one has to question whether nurse learners are currently provided with appropriate opportunities and means to develop such skills.

Over the last few decades, local wound treatment of established pressure sores has been one of the most controversial aspects of care. Studies have shown an enormous variety of preparations in use (David et al 1983), some with doubtful efficacy and others which contravene district policies on pressure sore management (Anthony & Dunn 1987). Rationale for dressing choice is often unclear or absent, and frequently guided by factors such as personal preference, ward preference (Sister's likes and dislikes) and tradition (Semple 1987). The proliferation of new primary dressings over recent years have added to, rather than resolved, the problem of product selection. As Thomas (1989) points out, dressings have now become more wound specific and this may limit their application to only certain types of wound. Selection of the most appropriate product can be extremely difficult.

THE RESEARCH PROBLEM

The nursing literature provides a rich source of information on the topic of pressure sore management, information which needs to be made available in a manner which is useful to, and immediately usable by, the practitioner. If current knowledge could be encapsulated within an expert system environment, perhaps nurses might be encouraged to adopt such a system as an aid to learning and problem solving. With these issues in mind, the main objectives of the research were:

1. To collate current knowledge from the literature on pressure sore risk assessment and wound management
2. To encapsulate that knowledge within an expert system environment
3. To evaluate the response of nurses to the system's content and potential as a decision support tool and learning aid.

SOFTWARE SELECTION

Following a review of the literature on both pressure sore management and expert systems, it was necessary to select the appropriate software to begin construction work. It had been decided to purchase an expert system shell, a ready-made program which was designed to assist the construction of an expert system (Barron 1989), and then to develop the knowledge base using its inherent facilities. It was the intention to develop the program at home using an existing Amstrad PCW 8512 machine. This decision would eliminate any hardware costs and ensure the equipment was accessible at all times. It soon became apparent that the majority of software applications available were designed for use on IBM PC type hardware, while the Amstrad used the older CP/M operating system. However, continued searching eventually revealed a product called WiseOne (Swallowsoft Publications) which had received a favourable review in the computer press (Davenport 1988) and was available for the Amstrad.

This package consists of two modules:

- the Knowledge Builder, which is used to construct the knowledge base
- the Consultant, which utilises the knowledge base along with user input data to draw inferences and recommend a certain course of action.

Within the WiseOne environment, knowledge is represented as a set of elements to which various values are attached, and a set of rules relating the defined elements. For example, in the context of pressure sore risk assessment, one might define 'ACTIVITY' as an element and assign it values such as 'fully mobile', 'walks with difficulty', 'chairbound', and 'bedfast'. Rules would then be written which explain how a certain action will be taken according to the identified value of 'ACTIVITY'. Such rules tend to follow an IF...THEN format, often referred to as a condition–action pair. Continuing with the above as an example, a rule might take the form:

IF: ACTIVITY is bedfast
THEN: pressure sore risk is HIGH.

The software attempts to arrive at some conclusion or goal through the adoption of a backward-chaining inference process. For example, when a primary goal is selected (e.g. 'identify risk status'), the program searches back through its rule structure to identify the first rule that must be satisfied in some way before subsequent rules can be considered within the decision-making process. It then prompts the user with an appropriate question to elicit some kind of response. Once some value has been assigned, the next rule in the chain is fired. This process is continued until the program eventually reaches the rule which relates directly to the primary goal. By now it will have gathered enough data to conclude its consultation by offering advice on the primary goal.

SOFTWARE DEVELOPMENT

Traditional software development models focus on sequential processes, such as specification, design, implementation and testing. This model has been likened to a waterfall, with results from one step forming the input to the next. As Born (1989) points out, this approach is non-iterative and requires full specification work to be completed from the outset of the project. For expert systems development, however, an iterative model or prototyping approach is more appropriate. An iterative model is cyclical and allows for gradual construction and testing of the prototype design. Born outlines three stages of the prototyping cycle: definition; construction; and evaluation.

The definition stage involves setting objectives for the prototype, deciding upon its scope, and outlining the criteria upon which it will be tested. The next stage, that of construction, involves knowledge acquisition and the gradual build up or revision of the prototype design. Initially, a bare skeleton may be built which concentrates upon only the essential feature of the knowledge base. The prototype is then measured for success against the criteria set out in the definition stage. A decision then needs to be made, based on the test results, whether to begin the cycle again or conclude prototype development.

When beginning construction work, Element and Rule files first had to be written individually as simple text files in ASCII format. Unfortunately, the software did not provide an integral text editor for this purpose, so separate word processing software had to be used. These files were then loaded into the Knowledge Builder for processing into a single Knowledge File. The Knowledge Builder examines the content and syntax of the files as it constructs the knowledge base. Any errors or omissions are reported back to the operator for alterations to be made to the appropriate file (Element or Rule). As a separate word processor needed to be used once again for this purpose, error-reporting necessitated a great deal of swapping from one software package to another, a process made more laborious by the lack of a hard disk. To some extent, knowledge base construction was hampered by this limitation of the expert system software.

Once an error-free knowledge build has been completed, the new file is simply loaded into the Consultant Module for testing. This is relatively straightforward and involves selecting a primary goal (e.g. Identify Risk Status), then answering questions derived from the knowledge base as prompted by the system. In order to follow the inference processes, a 'trace' facility is included within the Consultant Module for use during software development stages. Thus the designer is able to examine visually the sequence of events which led the system to reach its conclusions. Inference processes may also be directed to the printer if a permanent record is required. Such a facility is useful when a large number of rules come into operation, and allow the designer to trace their paths more accurately. As was discussed above, at each testing stage, the knowledge base is measured for success against the criteria set out in the definition steps of the prototyping cycle.

THE COMPLETED KNOWLEDGE BASE

Construction work continued in this cyclical fashion for approximately nine months, with each round of the cycle systematically elaborating upon the work of the previous design. On termination of development work, knowledge base consultation was available in two main areas:

1. Pressure sore risk assessment
2. Wound management (dressing selection).

Both these functions are encapsulated within the acronym PAWMEX (the **P**ressure sore risk **A**ssessment and **W**ound **M**anagement **EX**pert system).

The complete PAWMEX system occupies 167K of disk space. This figure takes into account not only the knowledge file, which is the basis of its reasoning, but also the various commentary files which support and enhance its decision-making capabilities. Reasoning within the knowledge file is based upon the following components:

45 Elements
67 Rules
146 Conditions.

SYSTEM OPERATION

Once a primary goal (e.g. Risk Status) is chosen, the system prompts the user with a relevant question and offers a number of alternative 'answers' or options to choose from. A typical response screen is illustrated in Figure 8.1.

The user responds by selecting the option which best fits the observed characteristics of the patient. If the user is unsure why the question is important or unclear as to which choice to make, the system can be asked for help. The help facility then provides the rationale for the inclusion of each element considered during the

122 NURSING INFORMATICS

```
┌─────────────────────────────────────────────────────┬──────────────┐
│ Subject: Pressure sore assessment and wound management │ WiseOne      │
│ ─────────────────────────────────────────────────── │ Expert System│
│ Action:      CONSULTATION on – $risk                │ CONSULT      │
└─────────────────────────────────────────────────────┴──────────────┘

   How have you assessed the patient's visual skin state (at risk areas)?
   Use the help facility for explanation and advice if required

   w  ... WHY?
   1  → intact
   2  → blanching hyperaemia
   3  → non-blanching hyperaemia
   4  → superficial damage
   h  ... HELP text
   m  ... return to menu

   Please choose an answer (NECESSARY question):  ■
```

Figure 8.1 Consultation on skin state.

```
┌─────────────────────────────────────────────────────┬──────────────┐
│ Subject: Pressure sore assessment and wound management │ WiseOne      │
│ ─────────────────────────────────────────────────── │ Expert System│
│ Action:      CONSULTATION on – $risk                │ CONSULT      │
└─────────────────────────────────────────────────────┴──────────────┘

   View more ... y/n?
   INTACT
   There is no evidence of reddening (erythema) and the skin surface remains
   unbroken

   BLANCHING HYPERAEMIA
   Following the release of pressure on the skin surface, a flow of excess blood into
   the affected tissues (reactive hyperaemia) causes a distinct superficial reddening
   of the area (erythema). Light finger pressure will cause blanching of this
   erythema, indicating that the microcirculation is still intact. At this stage, no
   damage has occurred.

   NON-BLANCHING HYPERAEMIA
   At this stage, the erythema remains when light finger pressure is applied. This is
   indicative of microcirculatory disruption and inflammation. If sensory innervation

   View more ...y/n?   ■
```

Figure 8.2 Help screen on skin state.

assessment process, and detailed definitions of each of the element values which the user has to choose from. Figure 8.2 illustrates one of the Help screens displayed if help is requested during consultation on the patient's skin state.

Thus, a detailed understanding of the topic can be gained, with all users sharing the same understanding of the terminology used. This latter issue is essential to ensure high inter-user reliability. All text files within PAWMEX are supported with references from existing publications, whilst a bibliography of over 100 articles and books provides suggestions for further reading. To facilitate simple up-dating as new research emerges, the text files containing this information exist separately from, and are called up by, the main knowledge file. They can thus be amended or added with a text editor or word processor, without alteration to the main program.

SYSTEM EVALUATION

From a software design perspective, it was felt necessary to obtain independent evaluation of such aspects as ease of use, content, and potential value. Arrangements were made for a small group of nurses to have access to the system, and a short operating booklet was compiled which assumed no previous computer experience. A brief questionnaire was constructed to elicit their views.

The total sample was made up of 12 nurses. This included four (33.3%) qualified practitioners, five (41.6%) students and three (25%) teachers. Of the staff within the clinical area, length of time qualified ranged from 1 to 15 years, whilst the level of experience of the students ranged from 5 to 36 months of training. The teaching staff had been qualified between 12 and 19 years. Because of the small sample size results must be treated with caution. However, it is likely that any major difficulties with the system would have emerged during testing by such a group.

Only seven (58.3%) of the sample indicated previous experience with computers or similar applications. Two (16.6%) had studied computing to 'O' level standard whilst at school, two (16.6%) were familiar with word processing, and three (25%) had had a short introduction to computers during a particular course of study. Three (25%) indicated that they actually owned a home computer. No respondent admitted having prior experience with expert systems.

Of the 11 questions contained in the questionnaire, the first three questions describe the study sample, while the other eight describe the reactions to the system. The results are presented in Table 8.1.

Table 8.1 Results of evaluation of PAWMEX

Question	Teacher (n = 3)	Qualified (n = 4)	Students (n = 5)	% of total
PAWMEX booklet easy to follow	3	4	5	100
System easy to operate	2	4	5	91.6
Difficult to operate	1	0	0	8.33
Terminology understandable	3	4	5	100
References useful for study	3	4	4	91.6
References not useful	0	0	1	8.33
Very useful decision support tool	2	2	2	50
Useful as decision support tool	1	2	3	50
Very useful learning aid	3	3	2	66.6
Useful learning aid	0	1	3	33.3
Would make changes/additions	2	1	3	50
Would not make changes/additions	1	3	2	50
Permanent installation	3	4	5	100

The results suggest that the PAWMEX system was well accepted by all concerned: this was supported by verbal feedback from a number of the sample. Their overall evaluation was very positive in terms of its content and its potential use as both learning aid and decision support tool. Furthermore, all respondents expressed the desire to see knowledge-based systems such as PAWMEX permanently installed within the clinical area.

Regarding the suggestions for changes to the system (Question 10), most were concerned with the way in which information was presented on the screen. Unfortunately, no facilities exist within the software used to alter the general screen format and allow for creativity of screen design and data presentation.

IMPLICATIONS FOR NURSING

Pressure sores remain a perennial problem for nursing, affecting between 4 and 10% of the various patient populations (Jordan & Clark 1977, Jordan et al 1977, Lowthian 1979, Ek & Boman 1982, David et al 1983, Nyquist & Hawthorn 1986, Semple 1987), and sometimes even contributing to patient death (Torrance 1983). The annual cost to the NHS as a result of increased hospital stays and additional treatments has been estimated to be in the region of £420 000 000, a figure which does not take into account further costs attributed to community care (Exton-Smith 1987). Whether the implications of pressure sore development are considered from the patient perspective or from that of the financial burden to the NHS, it is clear that the high incidence is unacceptable, particularly if it is accepted that approximately 95% of sores are probably preventable (Waterlow 1988).

Medical research has shown how expert systems can help improve doctors' diagnostic skills. As a result of this improved performance, de Dombal (1984) suggested that improved diagnosis could lead to savings of up to £100 000 per hospital per annum. Although no comparable data is available at today's prices, such savings are likely to be considerably higher, now and in the future. If similar results could be anticipated within the nursing domain of pressure sore risk assessment and management, the potential savings in terms of both unnecessary costs and reduced suffering are enormous.

Although initial financial outlay may cause some nurse managers concern, costs can be reduced by ensuring that expert systems are developed which are capable of integration with existing nurse management systems. For example, facilities such as those offered by PAWMEX might prove useful alongside a patient care-planning system and could facilitate the inclusion of important assessment and management data within the nursing documentation. Similarly, for those concerned with monitoring the quality of patient care, system consultation may form a component of the audit process and be linked to an existing measurement tool. A recent report which examines the application of knowledge-based systems in health care concludes that expert system investment would probably prove to be cost-effective in the long term (CSS 1989).

CONCLUSIONS

Information technology can provide nurses with the means to develop powerful computer systems to aid decision making and assist the learning process. This chapter has summarised the work of one such project in the field of pressure sore risk assessment and wound management (Woolley 1990). At this stage, however, the work is by no means complete. PAWMEX has not yet been tested in the clinical area for predictive accuracy or reliability. Such testing is essential if nurses are to plan care according to its recommendations. PAWMEX is also a 'stand alone' application developed on non-standardised hardware. Future work in this area needs to consider important issues such as hardware compatibility and system integration.

Pressure sore management is only one aspect of care in which expert systems can assist nurses. Nursing diagnosis (Hannah 1987) and care planning (Bloom et al 1987, Harrow 1988) have already received much attention and other problem areas such as pain assessment and management provide scope for further research. Expert systems provide valuable tools to aid decision making and facilitate learning; tools which current and future practitioners should consider if patient care is to benefit from that which IT has to offer in this fascinating area of computer science.

REFERENCES

Anthony D, Dunn A 1987 Keeping up to date on treatments. Nursing Times, 2 September, 42–44

Barron R 1989 Great expectations. Systems International, April 1989, 35–40

Barton A, Barton M 1981 The management and prevention of pressure sores. Faber & Faber, London

Bloom K C, Leitner J E, Solano J L 1987 Development of an expert system prototype to generate nursing care plans based on nursing diagnoses. Computers in Nursing 5(4): 140–145

BNF 1989 British National Formulary: 17. British Medical Association & The Royal Pharmaceutical Society of Great Britain, London

Born G 1989 Back to the drawing board? Systems International April 1989, 31–34

Braden B, Bergstrom N 1987 A conceptual schema for the study of the aetiology of pressure sores. Rehabilitation Nursing 12(1): 8–12, 16

Burnard P 1987 Towards an epistemological basis for experiential learning in nurse education. Journal of Advanced Nursing 12: 189–193

CSS 1989 Benefits and risks of knowledge based systems. Oxford University Press, Oxford

Davenport D 1988 Micro sapiens. Computing with the Amstrad PCW, January, 12–16

David J A, Chapman R G, Chapman E J, Lockett B 1983 An investigation of the current methods used in nursing for the care of patients with established pressure sores. Nursing Practice Research Unit, Middlesex

de Dombal F T 1984 Clinical decision making and the computer: consultant, expert, or just another test? The British Journal of Health Care Computing 1(1): 7–13

de Tornyay R, Thompson M A 1987 Strategies for teaching nursing, 3rd edn. John Wiley, New York

Ek A C, Boman G 1982 A descriptive study of pressure sores: the prevalence of pressure sores and the characteristics of patients. Journal of Advanced Nursing 7: 51–57

Exton-Smith N 1987 The patient's not for turning. Nursing Times, 21 October, 42–44

Gebhardt K 1987 Pressure points. Nursing Times, 15 July, 34–35

Goldstone L A, Goldstone J 1982 The Norton score: an early warning of pressure sores. Journal of Advanced Nursing 7: 419–426

Gosnell D J 1987 Assessment and evaluation of pressure sores. Nursing Clinics of North America 22(2): 399–416

Gould D 1985 Pressure for change. Nursing Mirror 161(16): 28–30

Gould D 1986 Pressure sore prevention and treatment: an example of nurses' failure to implement research findings. Journal of Advanced Nursing 11: 389–394

Hannah K J 1987 Understanding the concepts of computer based decision support systems for nursing practice. In: Hannah K J, Reimer M, Mills W C, Letourneau S (eds) Clinical judgement and decision making: the future with nursing diagnosis. John Wiley, New York

Harrow M 1988 A computer for clinical nursing. British Journal of Health Care Computing, January, 28–30

Holmes R, Macchiano K, Jhanhiani S S, Agarwal N R, Savino J A 1987 Combating pressure sores—nutritionally. American Journal of Nursing, October, 1301–1303

Jones J 1986 an investigation of the diagnostic skills of nurses on an acute medical unit relating to the identification of risk of pressure sore development in patients. Nursing Practice 1: 257–267

Jordan M M, Clark M O 1977 Report on the incidence of pressure sores in the patient community of the Greater Glasgow Health Board Area on 21st January 1976. University of Strathclyde Bioengineering Unit and the Greater Glasgow Health Board, Glasgow

Jordan M M, Nicol S M, Melrose A L 1977 Report on the incidence of pressure sores in the patient community of the Borders Health Board Area on 13th October 1976. University of Strathclyde Bioengineering Unit and the Borders Health Board, Scotland

Lowthian P 1979 Pressure sore prevalence: a survey of sores in orthopaedic patients. Nursing Times, 1 March, 358–360

Luckman J, Sorenson K C 1980 Medical-surgical nursing: a psychophysiologic approach. W B Saunders, Philadelphia

Merchant J 1989 The challenge of experiential methods in nursing education. Nurse Education Today 9: 307–313

Munro M F 1982 Analysis of problem solving strategies in nursing using written simulations of clinical situations. In: Henderson M S (ed) Nursing education. Churchill Livingstone, Edinburgh

Norton D, McLaren R, Exton-Smith A N 1962 An investigation into geriatric nursing problems in hospitals. Churchill Livingstone, Edinburgh

Nyquist R, Hawthorn P J 1987 The prevalence of pressure sores within an area health authority. Journal of Advanced Nursing 12: 183–187

Pajk M, Craven G A, Caerson-Barry L 1986 Investigating the problems of pressure sores. Journal of Gerontological Nursing 12: 11–15

Reichel S M 1958 Shearing force as a factor in decubitus ulcers in paraplegics. Journal of the American Medical Association 166(7): 762–763

Semple M J 1987 Theory and practice—a sore point? An investigation into nurses methods of management of pressure sores. Unpublished Diploma in Nursing Dissertation, University of Wales, Cardiff

Thomas S 1989 The dressing times. Welsh Centre for the Quality control of Surgical Dressings, Bridgend

Torrance C 1983 Pressure sores: aetiology, treatment and prevention. Croom Helm, London

UKCC 1986 Project 2000—a new preparation for practice. United Kingdom Central Council, London

Vasile J, Chatin H 1972 Prognostic factors in decubitus ulcers of the aged. Geriatrics, April, 126–129

Versluysen M 1986 Pressure sores in patients admitted for hip operations. Geriatric Nursing, March/April, 20–22

Waterlow J 1987 Calculating the risk. Nursing Times, 30 September, 58–60

Waterlow J 1988 Prevention is cheaper than cure. Nursing Times, 22 June, 69–70

Woolley N N 1990 Development of an expert system prototype to assist pressure sore risk assessment and wound management. Unpublished MN thesis, University of Wales, Cardiff

Woolley N 1992 PAWMEX—an expert system prototype. Information Technology in Nursing 4(1): 5–7

9

Computers' use for professional practice: what do nurses need to know?

S. Grobe

Introduction	3. Nursing science approach
Is it true?	a. Nursing practice in the future
1. Content approach	b. Technological innovations
Clinical applications	c. Nursing phenomena data
2. Competencies approach	Preparing practitioners for future practice

INTRODUCTION

What do nurses need to know about computers—and about computers' use for professional practice? A vexing question, yet one that demands critical analysis of the present and a view towards the uncertain future.

First, let us briefly examine the present and what we know about technology's place in today's health care scene. Automated information systems and automated care technologies are gradually becoming commonplace in health care settings (Saba & McCormick 1986). Increasingly, nurses are being involved in decisions about those systems (Zielstorff et al 1988).

Prospective payment systems, combined with diagnostic related group (DRG) automated systems, provide an example of technology's use in today's health care settings. Selected patient care information is combined with cost information and DRG rules, and an agency's reimbursements are calculated. Nurse staffing and scheduling systems provide a second example. Selected patient information (often in the form of acuity ratings), census, staff mix, and budgetary allocations are combined to yield a weekly or monthly staff schedule for nursing personnel (Ozkarahan 1987). Order entry and processing systems provide a third example. Selected therapies are processed; supply, inventory, and billing functions are handled automatically. Automated care delivery technologies provide additional examples. Automated intravenous infusion pumps for fluids and drugs (especially patient-controlled pain devices), ambulatory peritoneal dialysis technologies, urinary impedance devices, and laser-based treatment therapies exist in institutional and home care settings. Other technologies, such as computerised axial tomography, nuclear magnetic resonance and ultrasound, serve useful diagnostic functions.

Decision support technologies are being discussed in nursing conferences and in nursing research publications. For example, a microcomputer-based support system for nurse administrators has been tested (Brennan 1986), while database designs to support intervention modelling have been examined (Graves 1986). Guidelines for software development and selection for nursing administration expert systems were provided by Schultz (1984). Reasoned consideration for selecting appropriate nursing problems for expert systems have been explored by many nurse scientists.

And finally, electronic indexing, storage and retrieval functions provide very different but important examples of automated information handling. An automated system that allows quality assurance monitoring, whereby selected patient information is abstracted electronically, was described by Barhyte (1987). Nursing knowledge, stored as professional literature, is the second example: internationally available health professions literature is indexed, stored and retrieved through computer-based methods from the National Library of Medicine (Colaianni 1987, Sinclair 1987).

IS IT TRUE?

Now you ask: is it true? Are all these examples really in existence? How widespread are they? And, importantly, what if there are only a few examples of such technologies in the local area where you teach? How concerned should you be? And how do you determine what your nurses need to know about computers?

In today's information-intensive environment there is true cause for concern if nurse faculty find these examples of computer use in health care and nursing new or surprising. Conferences at international and national levels have been replete with information about technology and its effects on nurses and nursing. Many of the presentations from these conferences are being described in nursing literature. Further, assuming the responsibility for preparing professional practitioners demands that faculty continually keep one foot in the future—in that time period where those being prepared will practice. The other foot should be continually in the larger arena of professional practice—outside the local area of care through nursing's literature and its conferences.

This notion of faculty awareness, extending both into the future and beyond the local practice area, provides the framework for my attempt at responding to the question of what professionals need to know about computers for practice—the original question posed for this chapter.

Stated very simply, nurses first need to know about the present; second, they need to know how to continually adapt to the future; and they must know how to adapt in a deliberate, reasoned, and scientific manner. Thus the focus of this chapter centres on how to prepare today's students for an uncertain future that will be drastically influenced by advances in informatics.

I will use three alternative approaches in describing what practising nurses need to know about computers. Each approach has particular advantages and represents the time dimension of present or future. Some magical combination of all three approaches is most likely the best way to answer the original question. Two of the three approaches have already been discussed and analysed and are currently in the nursing literature. They are based primarily on the present, and I shall provide only an overview of them. The third, proposed in this chapter, relates to the uncertain future. The synthesis of all three approaches provides a comprehensive view of what nurses need to know about informatics for professional practice.

1. CONTENT APPROACH

The first approach is illustrated by Ronald & Skiba (1987). They provide computer content guidelines, thoughts on how to incorporate the content, and sample exercises in nursing curriculum based on detailed analysis of available faculty and institutional resources.

For example, one section of their current outline includes the application of computers to nursing. In abbreviated format the nursing applications include:

Clinical applications

1. Physiological monitoring
2. Documentation of the nursing process
3. Health care information systems
4. Decision support systems
5. Impact of clinical application.

Other topics included by the authors are: administrative applications; educational applications; research applications; and communications. The role of the nurse in selection, development, planning for implementation, and evaluation of the system is included and professional issues related to the use of computers in health care are discussed.

The overriding conceptual organising framework for Ronald & Skiba's ideas is based on a computer education continuum. Three levels of 'user competence' range from informed user through proficient user to developer. The user levels are bounded by two components representing types of kinds of knowledge and skill—a cognitive component and an interactive component. The cognitive and interactive components increase in size as a user moves along the continuum toward developer status.

2. COMPETENCIES APPROACH

A second approach to determining what practising nurses need to know about computers is represented in the proceedings from an international working group (Peterson & Gerdin-Jelger 1988). Nurse administrators, practising nurses, nurse educators, and nurse researchers met in a working group format in Sweden for the purpose of defining informatics competencies for nurses. A consensus technique was used by this select group of international representatives. The group first defined the basic information functions of nurses in the four roles (practice, administration, education and research). Next, specific examples of competencies for each information function across three levels of competence were defined.

The practising nurse has four information functions that imply informatics competencies. These include:

1. Documenting nursing practice
2. Accessing information
3. Using data and information of a system
4. Co-ordinating information flow.

Within the information functions of documenting nursing practice three examples of the different levels of competencies include:

a. Level I: knows the type of system in use
b. Level II: analyses the system in use
c. Level III: participates in designing and developing systems serving as an innovator of systems.

This competency approach represents an attempt to determine nurses' current information functions by their specific role, and then to create examples of the three levels of competencies from the simplest everyday use of computers to the more complex and innovative aspects of competence such as program development. This competency approach relies heavily on representing the current information functions for each nurse role. Thus it is primarily based on the present. The use of the consensus technique by a group of international nurses contributes a great deal of integrity to the competency statements recommended.

3. NURSING SCIENCE APPROACH

The third approach, the nursing science approach, requires future forecasting. As such it has no firm criterion standards against which it can be judged. Since assumptions underlie the projected future, the logic of the reasoning becomes a primary consideration. Thus, marked speculation can be dismissed, while reasoned conjectures can be considered.

Three aspects of the future must be considered before any projection of how to prepare practitioners can be proposed. The first aspect concerns defining the context of the nursing practice arena for the future. The second aspect concerns predicting the nature of determining what data represent nursing phenomena; and the third describes the potential methods for storing, retrieving, and communicating nursing data. Only after these three aspects of the future have been considered can we describe how to prepare nurses for this computer-based future.

a. Nursing practice in the future

The nursing practice arena for the year 2000 will be dramatically different from today's institutionally focused practice settings. Increased primary care environments and self-care oriented models are likely to predominate (Oberst 1986, NCNIP 1987, DeBack 1991). The nature and kind of nursing tasks will be altered drastically by these changes in practice environments (Kane et al 1986). The complexity of care will increase as it becomes information-laden and technology-driven (Stevenson & Woods 1986). The advent of clinical practice guidelines (Raskin & Maklan 1991) and implementation of the Institute of Medicine's recommendations for an automated patient record will demand increased attention to defining the critical data for nursing documentation systems of the future. Evidence supporting outcomes of care as related to nursing service provided will become increasingly important (Moritz 1991).

b. Technological innovations

The nature of the technological innovations that can be expected has the potential to alter the fundamental ways that nursing care is practised. For example, miniaturisation of electronic components, such as power sources and storage devices, as well as digitisation of data, may soon allow pacemaker or insulin pump implantation and regular status monitoring by phone from anywhere that has a telephone service. Similarly, signal processing advances may soon allow monitoring of vital physiological functions via satellite transmission from almost anywhere in space (Brand 1987).

In addition, information storage will have advanced to the stage where up to 800 pages of information can be stored magnetically on media that is the size of a bank credit card. The card can be read quickly by laser technology without ever wearing out. Thus, individuals may carry their entire health and medical history with them each time they present for care. The technology thus forces us to ask: are interviewing skills or data scanning and synthesising skills paramount in this nursing future?

These few technological innovations also illustrate the potential for serendipity that exists in any futuristic projections when technological inventions outstrip society's attempts to control or legislate for them (Brand 1987). It is important to recognise that the directions that technological inventions will take are unpredictable at best; the questions we ask now may be the wrong ones entirely. Only continual research and development with the available technological innovations will allow us to keep up to date.

c. Nursing phenomena data

The third aspect of the future that must be considered is determining what data are useful for representing and studying nursing phenomena. An initial step in this direction is represented by the Nursing Minimum Data Set (Werley et al 1986). However, determining what data are essential for nursing investigations and how they are modelled is critical (Graves 1986). In fact, one of the topics identified as a potential priority for research support from the National Centre for Nursing Research at its 1988 priority setting meeting was 'identification of the data sets for meaningful nurse science'. In the same way it is essential that we refine research methods that capitalise on examining nursing data in order to improve practice, generate knowledge and raise the quality of service utilisation (Fox & Ventura 1984, Oberst 1986). Finally, accessing available data from a variety of sources using communications technology, whether the data take the form of retrieved bibliographic citations or clinical data, is also an important aspect of any future nursing scenario (Anderson 1985, Sinclair 1987). Thus identifying nursing's care data and determining how such data might be used for improving practice and achieving better client outcomes is critically important.

PREPARING PRACTITIONERS FOR FUTURE PRACTICE

Consider the following few thoughts about the environment in which today's learners will practice. Nurse clinicians of the future are likely to be practising in independent roles and diverse settings. The nature of nursing practice in the future is likely increasingly to be based on clinical research and development efforts. The impetus for practice improvement will probably be derived from a philosophy of practice that builds on research that represents nurses' accumulated experience, as well as the eventual testing of nursing interventions in a more reasoned and deliberate manner than currently occurs. Accumulated experience and deliberative testing are based on comparisons that depend on reliable data. When data are aggregated in unique ways and in different patterns, information results. Replications of experiments using different data increase confidence in findings that have been proposed.

Computers are tools for accumulating and storing data. The nature of the data that are stored is a critical and overriding concern if we are to achieve the results that are necessary for scientific enquiry into practice. But how does this relate to our original question: what do nurses need to know about computers for professional practice? The answer is, I would suggest, that nurses need a view of the computer as a tool that is particularly useful for several reasons and for several purposes. Remembering that we are talking with the future in mind, and from the assumption that research about practice is the purview and responsibility of each practitioner, I would propose that nurses need to know that computers are:

- data machines
- information generators
- tools for practice that allow data collection for monitoring physiological parameters (perhaps in response to specific nursing interventions)
- tools for managing practice that allow data collection and analysis of phenomena associated with scheduling, costing, and evaluating outcomes of nursing services
- tools for accessing data for conducting research and for analysing and aggregating meaningful data for studying nursing's clients, clients' outcomes, and nursing strategies
- electronic tools for accessing information about clients in their care, and for obtaining the most recent and applicable research literature that can assist in determining the critical aspects of care
- useful tools for generating knowledge, especially by allowing the discovery of new perspectives on phenomena not recognised previously
- one form of technology that serves to sensitise us to dimensions of practice that we had not ever considered before and that
- the profession is in its infancy in determining what the data of nursing are, i.e. how they are characterised; what the data are useful for; and why selected subsets of data may be meaningful for examining practice.

Nurses also need to know about the impediments to greater use of automated systems. According to Zielstorff et al (1988) it is important that nurses and system vendors recognise what the barriers have been to clinically oriented nursing systems. These are also the factors that need to be described and discussed in preparing new professional nurses, especially since they may become part of the solution to the impediments.

First, the state of nursing knowledge is relatively undeveloped. The decision making of nurses and nursing vocabulary have received relatively little attention from nursing science, resulting in barriers to the development of systems that support clinical decision making. Second, the costs of developing the necessary software for clinical systems is great. On the other hand, there has been relatively little evidence generated to support the cost-effectiveness and cost benefits of these clinical decision support systems (Zielstorff et al 1988, p 33). Third, the user interface represents a continuing problem for clinical systems in that it requires data entry in a highly structured format; one quite unacceptable to clinical practitioners. For example, the rich narrative information of nurses notes or progress notes are not very accessible for retrieval and analysis. Therefore, interfaces that achieve a better cognitive fit with clinical users are necessary.

Finally, some user resistance exists when nurses are required to adapt to computer systems that are overly restrictive or difficult to use. Since adoption of computer systems is usually accompanied by dramatic changes, this also does little to comfort the users. Although these impediments seem overwhelming, their recognition is the first step towards a solution.

Nurses need to know that they are the thinking link between the definition of meaningful data and the meaning that may be derived from the data. Each nurse is critical and pivotal to this effort. Nurses who are prepared to be involved in computer systems development need to recognise the important part they play in analysing the vast spectrum of possibilities that exist, and must not be constrained by what vendors tell them about limitations on what is possible.

REFERENCES

Anderson Y 1985 Towards a nursing data base: a descriptive study. In: Hannah K J, Guillemin E, Conklin D N (eds) Nursing uses of computers and information science. Elsevier, Amsterdam

Barhyte D Y 1987 Computer-generated quality assurance: non traditional uses of the data. Journal of Nursing Quality Assurance 1(4): 43–49

Brand S 1987 The media lab: inventing the future at MIT. Viking Penguin, New York

Brennan P F 1986 Field test of a microcomputer based decision support system. In: Salamon R, Blum B, Jorgenson M (eds) Medinfo 86. Elsevier, New York

Colaianni L A 1987 Information services for the nursing profession from the National Library of Medicine. Journal of Professional Nursing, November/December: 372–375

DeBack V 1991 The national commission on nursing implementation project. Nursing Outlook 39(3): 124–127

Fox R N, Ventura M 1984 Efficiency of automated literature search mechanisms. Nursing Research 33, 174–177

Graves J 1986 Design of a database to support intervention modelling in nursing. In: Salamon R, Blum B, Jorgenson M (eds) Medinfo 86. Elsevier, New York

Kane M, Kingsbury C, Colton D, Estes C 1986 A study of nursing practice and role delineation and job analysis of entry level performance of registered nurses. National Council of State Boards of Nursing Inc, Chicago

Moritz P 1991 Innovative nursing practice models and patient outcomes. Nursing Outlook 39(3): 111–114

NCNIP 1987 National Commission of Nursing Implementation Project. Report of second invitational conference. NCNIP, Milwaukee

Oberst M T 1986 Nursing in the year 2000: setting the agenda for knowledge generation and utilisation. In: Sorenson G E (ed) Setting the agenda for the year 2000: knowledge development in nursing. ANA (The Academy), Kansas City

Ozkarahan I 1987 A flexible nurse scheduling support system. In: Stead W M (ed) Proceedings of the eleventh annual symposium on computer application in medical care. IEEE Computer Society Press, Los Angeles

Peterson H, Gerdin-Jelger U 1988 Nursing informatics competencies. National League for Nursing, New York

Raskin I E, Maklan C W 1991 Medical treatment effectiveness research. Evaluation and the health professions, June 1991, 14: 161–186

Ronald J S, Skiba D J 1987 Guidelines for basic computer education. NLN, New York

Saba V K, McCormick K A 1986 Essentials of computers for nurses. J B Lippincott, Philadelphia

Schultz S 1984 Languages, DBMSs, and expert systems: software for nurse decision making. Journal of Nursing Administration 14(2): 15–24

Sinclair V G 1987 Literature searches by computer. Image 19(1): 35–37

Stevenson J, Woods N F 1986 Nursing science and contemporary science: emerging paradigms. In: Sorenson G E (ed) Setting the agenda for the year 2000: knowledge development in nursing. ANA (The Academy), Kansas City

Werley H H, Lang N M, Westlake S K 1986 The nursing minimum data set. Journal of Professional Nursing 2(4): 217–224

Zielstorff R D, McHugh M, Clinton J 1988 Criteria for automated systems for nursing care planning. ANA, Kansas City

10

Information technology and the curriculum

M. Chambers

Introduction	The curriculum
Why information technology in a nursing curriculum?	Curriculum content
	Nursing
Science	Communication
Practice	Informatics
Management	Ethics
Research	Confidentiality
Education	Personal development
Participants in the IT experience	Teaching methods
Teachers and students	Student assessment
Attitude formation	Course evaluation
Anxiety	Summary
Planning the IT course	

INTRODUCTION

Information technology (IT) influences, directs and controls everyday life in a manner not previously imagined. Despite the obvious impact of IT on society it was not until the beginning of the last decade that it began to feature in nursing curricula, and even then most of the development was in America. However, by the middle of the 1980s some educationalists in the UK, especially those in institutions of higher education, were beginning to become active in the field of IT, a change which was also reflected in students' learning experiences (Chambers & Coates 1990). This development has continued at apace and seems destined to continue. As a consequence of this many nurse teachers are being very innovative in curriculum planning and using IT in many ways.

This chapter will:

1. consider some of the reasons why IT needs to feature in nursing curricula. It will focus on five major areas of nursing:
   - science
   - practice
   - management
   - research
   - education

2. consider a possible approach towards the integration of IT into the curriculum, and ponder some of the issues and difficulties which confront educationalists.

WHY INFORMATION TECHNOLOGY IN A NURSING CURRICULUM?

Science

The culture for the development of nursing as a scientific discipline has already been established. However, there is still a long way to go before it can be recognised as such. Indeed, some critics would suggest that this is not possible and indeed should not be part of any nursing agenda. Hayne (1992) quotes Sleicher, who suggested that nursing does not have a sufficiently 'well defined and well-organised body of knowledge' to be considered a discipline.

Bronowski (quoted in Smith 1981) tells us that

Science finds order and meaning in our existence. It is not a set of findings but a search for them. Human search and research is a learning by steps of which none is final and the mistakes of one generation are rungs in the ladder, no less than their correction by the next.... What science has to teach us is not its techniques but its spirit: the irresistible need to explore.

IT can make a valuable contribution to the journey of exploration by acting as a guide and a challenge. It can help find order and meaning in the confusion of theories and models which currently abound in nursing, some of which do nothing to ease the journey, but only add greater entanglement and enlarge the snare. Fitzpatrick (1988) stated that 'in developing nursing science the most pressing need is for conceptual clarity in identifying the phenomena of concern'. Here she believes that IT and computer technology in particular will assist 'not only in the developing of our science but also in enhancing nursing practice'. She also suggests that, at a level of conceptual analysis, 'computer technology could be applied to a content and context analysis of the nursing paradigm as reflected in the conceptual models of nursing'. Computer technology, she suggests, could thus help answer several questions regarding 'the basic components of nursing models, consistency across models and levels of congruence within models plus numerous other elements'.

In a similar vein Graves & Corcoran (1989) suggest that 'because nursing informatics deals with the rules and processes that operate on symbolic representations of nursing phenomena, nursing informatics is a legitimate area of study in nursing science'. The aim of nurse education is to prepare for the future, so if we are going to prepare nurse theorists and scientists who will further advance the science and theory of nursing it is imperative that they have a solid knowledge of computer technology.

Practice

IT has enhanced patient care in a variety of ways, including computerised clinical nursing systems and monitoring equipment as well as automated decision support systems. According to Warnock-Matheran (1988), while decision support systems follow very specific rules in solving problems, expert systems attempt to incorporate the experience and rules-of-thumb employed by the human expert. For example, the development of a microcomputer-based expert system to provide support for nurses caring for AIDS patients was described by Larson (1988), who claimed that 'the expertise of clinical nurse specialists in AIDS care could be captured and distributed in an easy, cost-effective, and timely manner to nurses and students who are less than expert, but who so desperately need the consultation and decision support of AIDS nursing experts'.

The development and utilisation of expert systems within nursing is not without its critics. Benner (1984) would seem to suggest that nursing practice has not been and cannot be formalised to the extent necessary for building an expert system. It has been suggested by others that perhaps only those specific elements of nursing where conceptual models have already been developed are amenable to expert systems. Again if either of these positions is to be advanced then the nurse of the future needs to have much more than a cursory knowledge of IT.

Management

Nurse management has changed greatly in recent years in the UK, influenced by a variety of factors including National Health Service (NHS) reforms, implementation of new nursing curricula (for example the Project 2000 programmes) and quality assurance initiatives. Many nurses, and more particularly senior nurses, hold positions for which an understanding of IT is essential. Fouchtman states that in the past 'nursing quality assurance activities were planned and organised by administrators. However, with continuing professional development and the increasing adoption of accountability-based or shared-governance practice models, quality assurance functions become an integral component of the role of the staff and individual practitioners'. Fouchtman also points out that the focus is now changing from quality assurance to continuous quality improvement. 'The collection of pertinent clinical information in order to measure this quality requires a familiarity with data collection methods and analysis. Practitioners must be proficient managers and interpreters of clinical information' (Fouchtman 1991). It is inevitable that as such initiatives move forward nursing will play a major role; indeed it is essential in order for nurses to influence the decision-making process with regard to the nature and quality of care delivery. As nursing more clearly identifies what information is required in order to make such informed decisions, nurse managers will increasingly be called upon to advise on decision support systems. In order to meet this requirement a sound knowledge of both hardware and software is critical if proper evaluations are to be made.

Research

For many people research and IT have always been closely linked, especially in the area of data analysis and statistics. As the number of nurses involved in research increases, so too will the demand for technological sophistication. Increased user competence will also lead to a more critical approach and better articulation of user requirements. Hence educationalists must be prepared and have an established firm foundation of IT and informatics in all basic nursing programmes so that higher-order skills can be more easily and appropriately developed.

Evidence of this development currently exists, with many nursing research projects utilising both quantitative and qualitative methodologies. This shift is a reflection of (a) the increased awareness in nursing of the need for a range of research strategies to answer complex questions, and (b) greater acceptance in the scientific community of the ethnographic or 'soft' approaches to research and the supporting literature.

It is important when introducing students to research that they are exposed to a range of methods and that they appreciate the potential of computer technology in helping to both analyse and write up their work. In addition the quality of work can be strengthened if individuals are capable of performing electronic literature searches and can use the technology to access, store and retrieve biographical material.

Education

For some time IT has played a part in nurse education at all levels but more especially in basic, post-basic and undergraduate education, largely through the use of computer-assisted learning (CAL) packages (Chambers & Coates 1990). Steele (1988) suggests that 'not only have traditional training programmes militated (albeit unconsciously) against the concept of information and how it might be applied to nursing; but they have also passively impeded the development of computer literacy or familiarity with the concepts and objective associated with information technology'.

Since both the above papers were written much has changed within nurse education, not least because of Project 2000. Students now use IT for a variety of reasons including preparation of assignments, analysis of data and care planning.

Although the use of CAL packages does still feature highly in the range of student activities, their scope and quality has improved considerably over the years. Many nurse teachers are now developing their own packages using authoring systems, an indication of just how confident, competent and adventurous teachers have become. Some teachers are also developing and using interactive video, as described for example by Eaton (1991). It is still early days in the development of IT in education, with endless possibilities not yet realised.

So far the discussion has concentrated on how IT has been used, and will continue to play a major part in nursing as a medium for generating and disseminating information and knowledge. It must be stated, however, that if IT is to be exploited to its full potential not only must nurses know how to operate the technology, they must also know something about how the technology actually works. This is not to say that everyone must become a computer 'whiz kid' but a working knowledge of the technology, at least to the extent of being able to distinguish between, for example, 286-, 386- and 486-based systems and to appreciate the memory requirements of modern applications software, is important to facilitate analysis and evaluation of both software and hardware systems and to articulate the needs of nursing to computer experts. Educational experience must prepare students to be able to use computerised care-planning systems, and input, store and retrieve data from ward-based terminals. Thus in addition to looking at the professional, ethical and legal implications the curriculum must also enable students to use computers as a vehicle for learning, equip them with the skills to utilise the technology in daily practice irrespective of setting, and give them an insight into how the technology works.

It has already been pointed out that many nurse education programmes do include IT as part of the curriculum (Chambers & Coates 1990, Eaton 1991). However, despite this there is a dearth of literature addressing the issues and problems. Many teachers speak of the need to include IT in the curriculum but to date little has been published either in relation to instigation or evaluation. Both are crucial elements if knowledge is to be shared and individuals prevented from 'reinventing the wheel'.

The contents of this chapter are based on personal experience of:

- attempting to introduce IT into curricula
- participating in the education track at the First European Summer School of Nursing Informatics in Holland in August 1991.

What follows therefore are not my thoughts alone but also reflect the experience of working with Professor Susan Grobe, of the University of Texas, the leader of the education track at the Summer School, and with other participants of the track.

PARTICIPANTS IN THE IT EXPERIENCE
Teachers and students

Before beginning to look at the curriculum it is important to give some consideration to those involved, i.e. the teachers and students.

Many of the current generation of nurse teachers were educated in an era when IT was confined more to science fiction texts than nurse education and practice. That has obviously changed and a great many teachers are very enthusiastic about becoming part of and indeed influencing the change. However, not all teachers share this enthusiasm. Among those who are keen the levels of skill and areas of interest are diverse; this is an asset rather than a hindrance as it should facilitate dissemination of knowledge. In an effort to establish a firm baseline of skills amongst teachers the English National Board for Nursing, Health Visiting and Midwifery (ENB) introduced the CAL project (Proctor 1988). This was aimed at providing a cohort of teachers with basic skills which they would share with colleagues. However, the number of teachers who successfully completed the programme during its 3-year existence was small. It is difficult therefore to assess the value of this project although evaluation data was collected throughout.

Students, on the other hand, are coming from a background where IT is commonplace. Large numbers of students are very familiar with computer technology and some know much more in this area than their teachers. There are also those who have little or no interest and have no desire to become knowledgeable let alone expert; not infrequently students ask the question 'what has IT got to do with nursing anyway?' This suspicion is similar in many ways to that expressed in relation to psychology and sociology in the curriculum. Students ask 'Why do we need to know about these subjects? We came here to learn about nursing.' These doubts do decrease, however, after clinical placements where students can more clearly see the relevance; some, however, remain sceptical.

Attitude formation

Developing a positive attitude towards IT is important. This is more likely to happen if students see its relevance and are taught by enthusiastic teachers. Fouchtman (1991) states, in relation to introducing Baccalaureate nursing students to research and computer concepts, that 'there is no consistent agreement on the sequences or content of educational experiences that are required to prepare baccalaureate nursing students for these varying experiences'. However she goes on to argue that 'there is consistent agreement on the importance of developing positive attitudes and enthusiasm for research and computer technology during the educational process'. Fouchtman is also of the belief that 'positive attitude development during initial education promotes the students' willingness to continue their future development and use of learned skills in their practice and also prevents later having to undo negative attitudes'.

Anxiety

Anxiety is closely related to attitude formation in that a little anxiety in a given situation is more likely to foster a positive attitude than is a situation which is highly charged with anxiety. Initially some teachers and students experience anxiety but with exposure, support and encouragement this disappears. A survey of computer literacy among undergraduates at University of Glasgow (Jones et al 1991) revealed that for 'one in four students the idea of working a computer makes them anxious'. It was also noted that those who had used a computer in the last month were less likely to be anxious.

In order to keep anxiety to a minimum it is important that students are gradually introduced to new concepts so that they move progressively from the known to the unknown. By adopting this approach the students' repertoire of skills is being extended but anxiety is minimised. Allowing students to work in pairs can also help where the more experienced students help the less experienced. However, this requires careful monitoring in order to prevent the experienced students feeling neglected or used, a position which could result in a lowering of interest.

PLANNING THE IT COURSE

Before considering what the course content should be it is important to address a number of key questions, for example:

- Are the physical and human resources sufficient and available to teach the course?
- Will the course be the sole responsibility of the nursing school or will responsibility be shared?
- Where in the overall curriculum will IT be taught?
- Will the IT component be taught as an integral part of other units, e.g. research, or will it be separate?
- What will be the title of the unit(s)?

Answers to some of the above will be influenced by the philosophy of the college and curriculum model being used. Individuals might say that some of the above questions, for example the unit title, are of little or no importance. However, the title given to any piece of learning or educational situation has the capability to shape and influence perceptions and expectations of what is to follow and consequently it can be important in shaping attitudes, especially if the subsequent experience does not meet expectations. For example, when this author first became involved with IT within the curriculum it was in connection with a unit entitled 'Care planning and Microcomputers'. Students remarked during evaluation that they found this title very anxiety-provoking and off-putting.

Combining two very different subject areas, although they were inter-related in this context, was problematic for both teachers and students. The nurse teachers had limited knowledge of computing and the students, with the exception of one (who had successfully completed an 'A' level course), knew little about either care planning or computing. Had it not been for the help given by two lecturers from the department of physics within the university it would have been impossible to achieve the unit objectives. The physics lecturers taught most of the computing elements while the nurse lecturers related the concepts to nursing and dealt with the care-planning aspects. Although the end result was satisfactory it was extremely anxiety-provoking for the nurse teachers concerned (Coates & Chambers 1989). In some instances the teachers were learning with and from the students.

Belenky et al (1986) state that 'when teachers and students are able to engage in the process of thinking together, talking about ideas and solving problems through public dialogue, personal and intellectual growth is readily achieved. A climate is created in which members of the class evolve their new and uncertain thoughts and nurture them safely to maturity'. This was indeed what happened in the above situation. However, it must be remembered that there were only 20 students in this class, and with larger classes this may be less feasible. Whether such an approach is desirable is another matter.

The curriculum

Many different approaches have been described regarding the teaching of IT to nurses (Ronald & Skiba 1988, Aarts 1989). As part of a doctoral programme at the University of Oregon, Bryson (1991) adopted a novel approach to investigating the perceptions of nurse educators regarding the type of IT experiences students on a degree programme should have in order to make them computer literate.

In order to develop her questionnaire Bryson used the Minnesota Educational Computer Consortium as a guide. This yielded some very interesting material which could act as a compendium for curriculum development.

For the education track at the European Summer School Professor Grobe organised the work into four sections reflecting major curriculum issues. These were:

- Informatics Competencies for Nurses: Definition and Related Factors
- Developing a Plan: Computer Integration in a Curriculum
- Preparing for Adoption: Organisational and People Factors
- Evaluation of Computer-assisted Learning.

Curriculum planning teams may wish to adopt a similar approach as it will help to focus and facilitate discussion about what exactly is to be achieved during the course, and thus will assist with the setting of objectives. It will also target the teaching methods to be used and suggest strategies to expedite integration. By drawing attention to organisational and people factors, practical and attitudinal issues will be highlighted and debated, helping the course to advance evenly and fairly.

An integral part of this process is the making of decisions about monitoring and evaluation of the course as well as looking at the integration and adoption of IT generally. Evaluation of CAL packages has absorbed much of the nurse educators' time in the past; it is an important area and requires attention, and there is an urgent need for some standardised measures for carrying out such evaluations. However, this must not be allowed to proceed to the exclusion of other considerations.

Ronald & Skiba (1988) point out the importance of establishing whether or not the computer component of the course is to be elective or compulsory. In the UK at present most IT components are an integral part of a diploma/degree programme and therefore compulsory. However, beyond a particular point there is no reason why IT should not be an elective.

Ronald & Skiba classify IT skills into three levels:

Level I: informed user
Level II: proficient user
Level III: developer.

INFORMATION TECHNOLOGY AND THE CURRICULUM 149

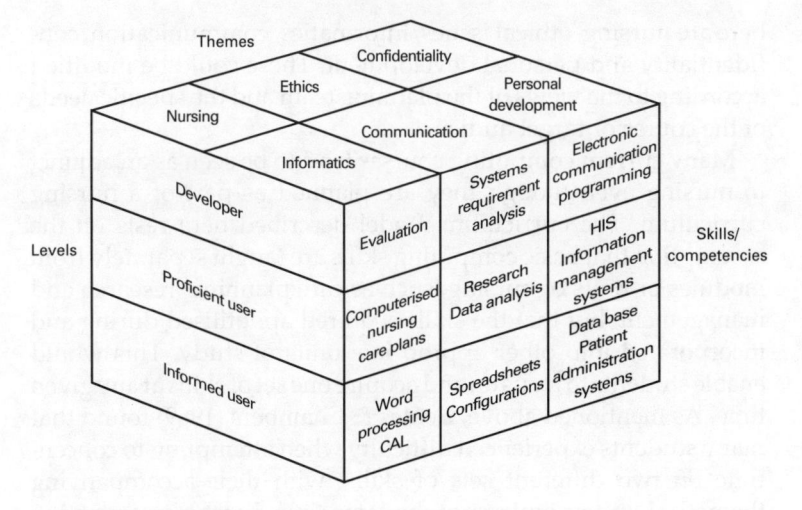

Figure 10.1 A curriculum model.

This classification provides a clear differentiation of the skills and knowledge requirements for each level. It could be suggested that these levels equate well with the different academic levels of current UK courses. For example:

Informed user = diploma level
Proficient user = degree level
Developer = postgraduate/masters level.

In this system Levels I and II would be compulsory as part of the programme. Level III, the developer level, could be an option for masters students. Completion of Levels I and II or equivalent would be a necessary entry prerequisite for Level III. Given the Credit Accumulation and Transfer System (CATS) currently being implemented in the UK, there is no reason why individuals could not take each level as a free-standing unit, with the associated assessment and accumulate credits for use at a later stage.

Curriculum content

A curriculum model which reflected this approach to the integration of IT would be developmental and progressive, with key themes running throughout (Fig. 10.1). Key themes suggested here are nursing, ethical issues, informatics, communication, confidentiality and personal development. These could be modified according to the views of the planning team and the specific needs of the course or target audience.

Many current computing courses tend to be seen as an adjunct to nursing even though they are planned as part of a nursing curriculum. The curriculum model described here rests on the assumption that basic computing skills are taught separately from modules or units of nursing, such as care planning, research and management, but that the skills acquired are utilised during and incorporated into other appropriate units of study. This would enable students to focus on and acquire one set of skills at any given time. As mentioned above, Coates & Chambers (1989) found that many students experienced difficulty when attempting to concentrate on two different sets of skills, with their accompanying theoretical underpinnings, at the same time. Learning computing skills as a separate but integrated unit should facilitate better understanding and enable students to analyse and synthesise subject matter more easily.

Ronald & Skiba (1988) appear to suggest that the skills of the informed user can be taught by anyone with a knowledge of IT. If IT is to become an integral part of nursing then nurse teachers with the appropriate skills must be available to ensure that this takes place. Depending on the IT skills of the teachers they can decide whether or not they wish to get involved in the theoretical aspects of IT. They must, however, be available to facilitate the students in relating theory to practice within a nursing framework.

Bryson (1991) believes that the primary responsibility of nurse educators is to teach nursing, and she questions whether or not nurse educators would be able to teach computing to a high enough level. However, she concludes by saying that until nurse educators become sufficiently qualified, holding for example a masters degree in computer technology, computing courses should be taught by computer specialists.

Irrespective of who teaches the course, if it is to be fully integrated into the curriculum all those involved need to make links from one unit to another. For example when introducing spread sheets it is necessary to draw students' attention to the parallels with computerised care planning or the production of duty rosters. When learning to use statistics packages it is important to use nursing examples and data, and in a research unit computing skills could be further enhanced if students enter, retrieve and analyse data as well as using word processing skills.

Planning for integration is very much a curriculum design and staff liaison issue. It is clear that units require to be developed in a congruous manner, with good communication and understanding between teaching staff. It could be suggested that the outcome of this integrated approach will therefore be to increase skills acquisition, reduce confusion and anxiety, increase motivation, facilitate students in anticipating problems, reinforce the relevance of computing to nursing and gradually take the student from the known to the unknown.

As has already been suggested, the issue of relevance is important in the context of attitude formation and the reduction of scepticism amongst students. The curriculum should be structured so that as well as students learning basic computing skills, they also have the opportunity to study and use IT in relation to all other appropriate units of learning. Simply linking subject matter to computers is insufficient: students must see it as having a useful contribution to make. IT must be put in context with its strengths, limitations and possibilities outlined from the beginning. Professor Grobe, in setting the scene for the education track at the First European Summer School of Nursing Informatics said 'We should be continually asking ourselves this question: How can informatics help improve the care that I give?' That question gave focus to the wide reaching debate that followed. It should also be at the forefront of the thinking of all nursing curriculum planners.

Each of the six themes within the outlined curriculum will now briefly be discussed, although it is not the intention to suggest specific content for each one. It is suggested that at the developer level, where students may be studying for a postgraduate diploma/masters course in nursing, other options should be available. For example if a nurse teacher is taking the course then it would be appropriate to examine IT more specifically in relation to the curriculum, education or research.

Nursing

Earlier in this chapter reference was made to the fact that currently a considerable number of IT courses are taught as an adjunct to nursing. The end result of this is that students have difficulty in seeing the relevance of IT to nursing. This difficulty is further compounded because not many students in the UK have the opportunity at present to see IT working in a meaningful way at ward level.

It is therefore essential that nursing as a discipline forms an integral part of any IT programme. Students must have the opportunity to see and understand how IT informs nursing and vice versa. The way in which IT can make a valuable contribution to the delivery of high-quality care and the development of nursing as a science, through enhancing the scope and quality of both the education and research processes, must be made explicit.

Not only must this connection be made explicit in the IT programme, it must be made explicit in all other components of the total curriculum, for example research, care planning, ethics and communication.

Communication

Communication is a vital component for a variety of reasons. IT provides a powerful medium for communication between individuals, departments and organisations. IT can also shape the form of communications, enhancing (or detracting from) their effectiveness, and enabling the creation and transmission of information in quantities and at levels of complexity not possible using more traditional means. Increasingly students must learn the skills of electronic communication in order to function on the wards.

Another important aspect of communication is the ability to construct and present an argument, when for example attempting to influence attitude formation, break down prejudices and inform decision-making processes. The disciplines associated with the processing of data and the use of computers for data analysis can greatly assist with the clarification of ideas and thought processes. Finally, electronic communication, via E mail, bulletin boards and conferencing systems can enable students to correspond with fellow students and other professionals all over the world, presenting excellent opportunities for debate and the exchange of ideas and experiences.

Informatics

This section of the curriculum will aim first to introduce students to the technological aspects of computing, how a computer works, its potential and limitations. Second, at developer level, students will be required to examine critically their thinking about nursing and to produce material that will be understandable to computer experts and which will succinctly reflect the particular area of nursing in which the work is being developed.

Critical thinking and analysis is an important skill to develop and occurs to a greater or lesser degree throughout the educational process of learning to nurse. Kintgen-Andrews (1991) discussed the findings from a number of studies concerned with critical thinking and nurse education in the USA, while Paul (1985) states:

> Most everyday thinking about pressing real-life problems crosses disciplinary categories and domains and involves opposing points of view and contradictory lines of reasoning....We need to ensure, therefore that students receive a substantial amount of practice in reasoning dialogically and dialectically, so that they become comfortable with and skilled in weighing, reconciling and assessing contradictory points of view through rational dialogue, discussion and debate.

Adequate knowledge of a subject area is vital in order to be able to critically assess its value and contribution and to make decisions about what to accept or reject from the information/knowledge presented.

In the past nursing has had little practice at differentiating the components of knowledge necessary for the completion of specific tasks. However, there is now considerable effort being channelled into the development of nursing minimum data sets and this means that decisions will have to be made by nurses about the nature of the data to be collected and the purposes for which it will be used.

Consequently a knowledge of IT is not only important as a means of facilitating development in IT, but in all areas of nursing: familiarisation with a disciplined mode of thinking will help refine and develop the science of nursing. Kintgen-Andrews (1991) argues that this is particularly true in the case of clinical decision making.

Ethics

So far courses which have attempted to introduce nurses to IT seem to have included little or nothing about ethics, although issues relating to confidentiality have been addressed. If we accept that ethics is associated with questions about morality, and morality is largely about deciding whether or not something is good or bad, then clearly there is much to discuss in relation to IT. Wainwright

(1991) pointed out that 'in general it seems as though it is taken for granted that the development of informatics is beneficial and desirable, and that all we need to do is take a few simple precautions with regard to security'. However, he goes on to argue that this is by no means a foregone conclusion, and by highlighting ethics as a theme within an IT module and by including a chapter in this text it is hoped that curriculum developers will give this element greater prominence.

Confidentiality

This section has links with ethical issues. However, its major thrust will be to look at the 1984 Data Protection Act and access to information in general, from a legal, practical and organisational perspective. The Data Protection Act was passed in order to allow the monitoring and control of personal information held on computer, by registering all non-exempt personal data systems in the UK (Bryant & Griffiths 1985). Although this has gone some way to protect the individual there is still potential for mishandling of data. Nurses handle large amounts of data daily and as technology comes closer to the ward a greater knowledge of the Act and its consequences is required.

Personal development

In all nursing courses emphasis should be placed on students' development of self-evaluation, allowing them to identify their own strengths and weaknesses and where possible working at their own pace to achieve their potential. This can be accomplished in a number of ways, but particularly through reflection in action and self- and peer assessment.

IT, like any other part of the curriculum, should be developed in this manner. Indeed IT itself, in the form of CAL and interactive video for example, can be of assistance in enabling students to achieve personal goals and interests through working at their own pace in relative privacy.

TEACHING METHODS

Clearly the best approach to the learning of skills is one that is primarily experiential. However, practice needs to be supplemented with supervision, both in the laboratory and in the ward environment. Gradually this supervision can be withdrawn as individuals become more confident. In the ideal situation students should have the opportunity to work with both mainframe and personal computer systems. Where possible they should have the opportunity to use in the laboratory the same patient information and care-planning systems that are operational in the clinical settings. It is recognised that this would be problematic in some instances because students have placements in different hospital and community settings which may be using different systems, although skills acquired on one system will probably be transferable.

Lectures, discussions and tutorials are also valid teaching methods. Paper-and-pencil and group problem-solving exercises may in many ways prove more important than practical sessions at the terminal, as students learn the skills and disciplines of problem identification and formulation, and come to understand the importance of proper planning. Group sessions and tutorials may also prove beneficial ways of examining attitudinal and other personal issues such as fear or anxiety.

STUDENT ASSESSMENT

Assessment is an integral part of any learning experience because it provides feedback for both teachers and students. Assessment methods should reflect the curriculum model, course objectives and content. The prime objective of most IT courses is one of skill acquisition, so assessment strategies must reflect this, although it is important that IT is firmly placed within the context of nursing. Assessments should be placed in an appropriate context, with opportunity for students to demonstrate their IT skills across a range of situations which reflect the course level. With this in mind, decisions will be reached at the planning stage as to how this is best accomplished. For example it may be agreed that in relation to informed user level the students will submit an essay in relation to a specified nursing unit, typed using a word processor. They might also demonstrate their competence in using CAL packages by evaluating such a package in relation to a particular unit.

For the proficient user, assessment might be by way of demonstrating competence in relation to the inputting and analysis of data using a particular statistical package, while assessment at the developer stage might involve evaluation of a nursing system or a specified contribution to the development of a nursing information or care-planning system.

COURSE EVALUATION

It is essential that all courses be evaluated, but this is especially true in the area of IT as it is so much at a developmental level. This evaluation can be both formative and summative and take whatever form the course planning team consider appropriate, although it is tempting to suggest that the method used might involve IT in some respect. For example, the design and construction of an interactive computer-based evaluation questionnaire and the analysis of the data generated would be an excellent project for students at an appropriate level of competence.

It is important that the outcomes of such evaluations are shared with colleagues and published in national and international journals. Sharing information, especially regarding the difficulties and problems experienced and how they might be overcome, will contribute to the development of better techniques and approaches and reduce the risk of others repeating one's own costly mistakes. There is a tendency for only the success stories to be published, but there is also a need (arguably a greater need) for the less successful experiences to be discussed in an open forum if a body of knowledge is to be established.

SUMMARY

This chapter has attempted to examine some of the reasons why an understanding of IT is important to nursing, and to show how IT and informatics might be integrated into the curriculum. The importance of good communication and liaison between teaching staff has been emphasised.

Significant emphasis has been placed on the importance of 'hands-on experience' as the major teaching method. One of the key problems to be faced in the successful introduction and integration of IT is the fact that not all teachers or students of nursing are totally convinced of the contribution of IT to nursing, and their concerns must be taken into account. It is important to remember that IT is there to facilitate the nurse in providing the best possible patient care, not to replace the nurse. By the same token, nurse education exists to produce competent nurse practitioners, not computer technicians.

Finally, to quote from a paper delivered by Matthews (1988) at the Third International Symposium on Nursing Use of Computers and Information Science, those interested in computers might well be classified along similar lines to Kenninstone's classification of drug takers:

1. 'The Tasters', who use them only occasionally, usually experimenting;
2. 'The Seekers', who use them regularly but not with any lifestyle built around them apart from a general search for relevance;
3. 'The Heads', that small but highly vocal minority who have a totally turned on ideology and for whom drugs, or computers, are the passport to their sub-culture.

We must beware that the sub-culture... of computing in nursing does not become an ideology in itself, a kind of marijuana to make the unseemly side of the job less offensive (Matthews 1988).

REFERENCES

Aarts J E C M 1989 A curriculum in nursing informatics. In: Salamon R, Protti J, Moehr J (eds) International Symposium of Medical Informatics and Education. University of Victoria

Belenky M, Clinchy B M, Goldberg N R, Tarule J M 1986 Women's way of knowing. Basic Books, New York

Benner P 1984 From novice to expert: excellence and power in clinical nursing practice. Addison-Wesley, Menlo Park

Bryant N, Griffiths G 1985 Caught in the act. Nursing Times 81(45): 16–17

Bryson D M 1991 The computer-literate nurse. Computers in Nursing 9(3): 100–107

Chambers M, Coates V E 1990 Computer training in nurse education: a bird's eye view across the UK. Journal of Advanced Nursing 15: 16–21

Coates V E, Chambers M 1989 Teaching microcomputing to student nurses: an evaluation. Journal of Advanced Nursing 14: 152–157

Eaton N 1991 Interactive video as a teaching medium. Nursing Standard 5(14): 31–36

Farabaugh N 1990 Maintaining student interest in CAL. Computers in Nursing 8(6): 249–253

Fitzpatrick J J 1988 Nursing: how do we know; what do we do; and how can we enhance nursing knowledge and practice. In: Proceedings of Nursing and Computers Third International Symposium. C V Mosby, St Louis

Fouchtman M M 1991 A nursing service-education model for introducing baccalaureate nursing students to research and computer concepts. Computers in Nursing 9(4): 152–158

Graves J R, Corcoran S 1989 The study of nursing informatics. Image: Journal of Nursing Scholarship 21(4): 227–231

Hayne Y 1992 The current status and future significance of nursing as a discipline. Journal of Advanced Nursing 17: 104–107

Jones R B, Navin L M, Barrie J Hillan E, Kinane D 1991 Computer literacy among medical, nursing, dental and veterinary undergraduates. Medical Education 25 191–195

Kintgen-Andrews J 1991 Critical thinking and nursing education: perplexities and insights. Journal of Nursing Education 30(4): 152–157

Larson D E 1988 Development of a microcomputer-based expert system to provide support for nurses caring for AIDS patients. In: Proceedings of Nursing and Computers Third International Symposium. C V Mosby, St Louis

Matthews J 1988 Nursing and computers—whither the next decade. In: Proceedings of Nursing and Computers Third International Symposium. C V Mosby, St Louis

Paul R W 1985 Critical thinking research: a response to Stephen Norris. Educational Leadership 42(8): 46

Proctor P 1988 We have the technology to rebuild... In: Proceedings of Nursing and Computers Third International Symposium. C V Mosby, St Louis

Ronald J A, Skiba D J 1988 Computer education for nurses: curriculum issues and guidelines. In: Peterson H E, Gerdin-Jelger U (eds) Preparing nurses for using information systems: recommended informatics competencies. National League for Nursing, New York

Smith J P 1981 Nursing science in nursing practice. Butterworth, London

Steele V 1988 Building UK nursing systems—bottom up. In: Proceedings of Nursing and Computers Third International Symposium. C V Mosby, St Louis

Wainwright P J 1991 Ethical implications of nursing informatics. Paper presented at the First European Summer School of Nursing Informatics. Leusden, The Netherlands

Warnock-Matheran A 1988 Expert systems: automated decision support for clinical nursing practice. In: Computers in Nursing Conference Proceedings Third International Symposium. C V Mosby, St Louis

11

The student nurse's use of information technology —A Welsh perspective

P. Chai Tin Tang

Introduction
Approach to the problem
Study questions
Methods
  The sample
Data collection
Survey results and discussion
  Students' knowledge of IT

Experience in the use of computers
  and present usage
Knowledge of facilities available
Formal educational opportunities
Organisation and teaching of IT
Attitudes of students
Students' expressed needs
Implications for nurse education
Conclusions and recommendations

INTRODUCTION

Good management depends on good information. Good information depends on good data which are relevant, valid, accurate, complete and timely. Good information is essential not only for those doing the principal work of the organisation but for those managing the organisation and related support services. Information is required to:

- establish objectives
- decide on policies to be pursued
- develop strategies
- arrange tactics
- agree targets
- monitor the plans and make necessary adjustments.

It has been stated that the National Health Service (NHS) has never been short of data but the provision of information at a time and in a format which managers and staff can use to base management decisions has been disappointing (Merrison 1979, Freeman 1990).

A number of significant events in recent years, such as the publication of the Griffiths Report (Department of Health and Social Security (DHSS) 1983) with the consequent introduction of general management, and the Korner Reports (DHSS 1984), with their concentration on minimum data sets, have highlighted the increased need for relevant, accurate and timely data to support health care management and planning.

With the prevailing political commitment to contain expenditure and obtain 'value for money' (HMSO 1989a), the need for information is further intensified. The White Paper brought into the public eye the growing pressure on the NHS to improve its resource management. For the NHS to manage its resources effectively, information about the availability and use of resources for patient care (money, time, people and equipment) must be provided on a disciplined basis. Information about each patient's need for health resources allied to information on resourcing has to be collected, stored, processed, analysed, aggregated and distributed. The volume and complexity of such information processing requires the use of IT.

It is unlikely that current objectives can be met without heavy investment in IT. As a consequence, computer-based information systems are being introduced very quickly to 'manage' the NHS in the same way that information technology systems are used in other sectors. This trend is expected to continue as the Government is prepared to provide some of the necessary finance for the information systems.

APPROACH TO THE PROBLEM

This information and computer revolution will change nursing practice (Schwirinan 1983). As resource management is implemented around the country, nurses, as a major source of activity data, have to take an increasing interest and involvement in promoting economy, efficiency and effectiveness whilst maintaining quality care. They are being forced to change and adapt working methods and behaviour to new technologies, expectations and demands.

The potential of computer-based IT in most areas of nursing, including administration, management, clinical practice, research and education, has been well documented in the nursing literature. The use of computer-based information systems in nursing to assist the nurse to organise and manage information is justified on grounds of efficiency, speed and cost containment. As the nursing profession becomes involved at the inception of these information systems, nurses become an integral part of systems development. If potential benefits are to be obtained, it is vital that as users, nurses become actively involved right from the start in defining the system specification so that the systems meet their needs as well as the needs of other staff and departments. Only if the right tool is selected by the organisation can there be any hope that the resulting information system will improve professional practice.

The nursing profession is urgently in need of people who can use technology effectively (Massie 1989). For IT to have a place in nursing, nurses must drive the computers, not vice versa; nurses must be making decisions about what the systems are to do (Melia 1990). What is needed are nurses who will adopt a proactive role, to use, direct and take a strong position in shaping automated systems that have an impact on their work. An understanding of IT and the implications of using IT (ethical, legal, social and political issues) is a necessity so that they can argue for their needs. Without an adequate understanding they will be left out of the debate, unable to participate because of their lack of knowledge, and they will become passive users of computer systems that have been developed for them by others. Without the involvement of knowledgeable nurses, information analysis, development, selection and implementation will be entrusted to the analysts and systems designers, who may not understand the basic needs of the users and the organisation in which they operate.

Too often nurses are presented with information systems without any involvement in the design and where little thought has been given as to what information is needed, by whom and how it will be used (Jarvis 1988, Fardell 1989).

Peel (1990) states that 'It is absolutely crucial that all health professionals should have detailed knowledge of, and certain competencies in information systems and information management.' Nurses must be 'computer literate'. This implies computer competency within the discipline plus an open awareness of technological possibilities yet unknown (Newbern 1985). However, when preparing future nurses for their role in an IT environment, several authors cite not only the need for computer-literate nurses, but also the need for the assumption of newly defined roles (Cox et al 1987). Anderson et al (1974) proposed three levels of preparation for all students and practitioners of health care disciplines. They propose that:

- the first level of preparation be a basic general level of computer education which provides a general knowledge of computers and data processing

- the second level of preparation be one in which people keep their main orientation as doctors, nurses, administrators but with the ability to take part and be involved in task analysis, design and implementation of systems.
- the third level of preparation be one which develops expertise in both health care delivery and computer science areas.

Ronald & Skiba (1987) also advocate a computer education framework consisting of a continuum of learning experiences. They believe that all nurses should be at the 'informed user' level, that most professional nurses should reach the 'proficient user' level, and propose a third 'developer' level for those who wish to pursue an advanced preparation. These levels of preparation clearly parallel those of Anderson et al (1974).

The Department of Health document 'A strategy for nursing' (HMSO 1989b) envisages a more highly computerised future for nursing and suggests that 'tomorrow's health care practitioners will need to use the computer with the same confidence that today's use the telephone'. This statement implies that tomorrow's nurses must acquire fresh knowledge and learn new skills. They 'must be equipped with the appropriate knowledge and skills to meet the needs' (Chapman 1974) and the ideal time to begin this process is during their basic nurse education programme (Andreoli & Musser 1985, Eaton 1987, Sultana 1990).

The majority of nurses have little awareness of the impact that IT will have on their work and future. The student nurses of today are the practitioners of tomorrow and will need to be confident, not only in their use of computers as personal tools, but also in their use as management tools to enhance their work. However, it is questionable whether they are adequately prepared to participate in an informed manner and to use information systems effectively.

STUDY QUESTIONS

This chapter reports a study that was undertaken to determine, from a Welsh perspective, the student nurse's attitude, knowledge and use of IT (with particular reference to the use of computers as a management tool) and the implications that this may have for nurse education. The study was conducted as part of a taught Master's degree programme.

The objectives of the study were :

1. To determine the students' knowledge of IT and the facilities that were available for their use.
2. To determine where the students have obtained their experience in the use of computers and their present usage of IT.
3. To enquire of the students what formal educational opportunities regarding the use of IT were available and who was responsible for the organisation and teaching of IT to them.
4. To determine the attitudes of the students towards IT.
5. To evaluate their current needs for education in IT and as a result to address the need for change in nurse education.

METHODS

The method of inquiry was a survey by questionnaire. To address the objectives of the study, the questionnaire comprised 64 questions and contained both open and closed questions. It was pretested with a group of 30 student nurses from one of the Colleges of Nursing and Midwifery in England. Some changes were made to improve the clarity of the questions and the amended questionnaire was used for the main study. Ethical approval was sought and gained prior to conducting the study.

The sample

The sample chosen for the study was student nurses from the seven Schools of Nursing in Wales (Clwyd, Dyfed, Gwynedd, Gwent, Mid Glamorgan, South Glamorgan and West Glamorgan Health Authorities) which at that time offered the 3-year basic nurse education programme leading to the Registered General Nurse qualification.

Because of time constraints it was decided that 10 student nurses from each year of the course from each of the seven Schools of Nursing would be invited to complete the questionnaire. This gave a total sample population of 210 subjects. The cohorts were chosen by convenience sampling and systematic sampling was used to select the 10 students from each cohort.

DATA COLLECTION

In each School of Nursing a link teacher was appointed by the Director of Nurse Education to assist with the study. The questionnaires were distributed to the subjects via the link teachers when the students were in school for a study period; the survey took place between 1 November 1990 and 10 January 1991. A letter of explanation was attached to every copy of the questionnaire to describe the survey instrument and to request participation. A return date for the completed questionnaire to the link teacher was specified.

The subjects were assured that participation in the study was voluntary and that they could withdraw at anytime. Confidentiality and anonymity were assured by coding the questionnaire in such a way that individual subjects were not identified but that identification was only by cohort and by School of Nursing. The questionnaires were returned to the researcher by the link teachers using the prepaid envelopes provided.

SURVEY RESULTS AND DISCUSSION

A total of 183 out of 210 questionnaires were returned, giving an overall response rate of 87.1%.

Responses were received from 57 (27.1%) first year students, 58 (27.6%) second year students and 68 (32.4%) third year students. Most of the respondents were in the 18–25 age range (67.2%), 15.3% were from the 34–41 age range and 14.2% from the 26–33 age range. The ages of the respondents may be important because many recent school leavers may come into nursing computer literate; the government's IT in Schools initiative means that more pupils now have exposure to computers within the curriculum, although the extent of this exposure is variable. Mature students are unlikely to have any experience of IT in primary or secondary education as they would have completed their education before computers were widely available. However, if mature students have had career experience in other areas before coming into nursing they may have had work-based experience of IT applications.

Students' knowledge of IT

62.3% of the respondents stated that they had been taught to use computers. Of these, 24% gained this knowledge prior to commencing nurse training and 25.1% during nurse training. However, only 35% of the study sample said that they would be able to set up (connect cables, etc) a computer, monitor and disk drive and slightly less than half (45%) would be able to load and run programs, suggesting that their competence is limited. 12% of the respondents claimed that they were able to develop programs.

Table 11.1 Confidence in using computers (n = 183)

Are you confident in using the computer for:

	Yes	No	No response
Word processing	59 (32.2%)	100 (54.6%)	24 (13.1%)
Data collection	30 (16.4%)	114 (62.3%)	39 (21.3%)
Spreadsheets	10 (5.5%)	121 (66.1%)	52 (28.4%)
Problem solving	21 (11.5%)	111 (60.7%)	51 (27.9%)
CAL	57 (31.1%)	87 (47.5%)	39 (21.3%)
Desktop publishing	8 (4.4%)	120 (65.6%)	55 (30.1%)
Games	89 (48.6%)	58 (31.7%)	36 (19.7%)

However, this area warrants further investigation, because at least two respondents thought that to develop programs meant to be able to work through a complete program without crashing it.

When asked if they were confident in using the computer for specified activities, the responses suggested that the respondents' confidence in using computers was low (Table 11.1). Only one-third of the study sample felt confident to use the computer for word processing (Table 11.1). Even for those respondents who have had some training or had attended a word processing course during training, only 50% felt confident to use computers to carry out this activity.

In the area of computer-assisted learning (CAL), it is surprising to note that less than one-third (31.1%) of the respondents were confident in using CAL packages (Table 11.1) even though this requires only an elementary knowledge of computers. Although CAL is an established educational tool, this may not have been fully recognised by nurse educators. The reluctance on the part of teachers to encourage the use of CAL in the Schools of Nursing surveyed may have hindered the efforts to increase computer literacy of nursing students.

When asked if they were able to define their requirements for a computer system and to argue for computer systems which would be of benefit to nursing, 88% of the respondents reported that they were not confident to define their requirements and 82.5% did not feel able to argue for systems of benefit to nursing. The main reasons given for their lack of confidence were their lack of knowledge and experience. The results show that the students' knowledge, poor as it is, is restricted to microcomputers for personal and educational use. This is an inadequate base for working with management information systems.

Experience in the use of computers and present usage

42.1% of the respondents entered nursing with computer experience. Of these, 57.1% gained this experience whilst in school or college through undertaking GCSEs, 'A' levels, basic computing or word processing courses or when computer use was integrated as part of a course. 42.9% gained their experience through work, in places such as banks, Department of Social Security, a doctor's surgery, chemist's shops, general stores, post offices, agricultural and horticultural forestry departments, local health authorities, florists, the vehicle registration office or the Royal Air Force. They reported computer experience in word processing, labelling systems, stock control, statistical analysis, and basic programming.

The respondents were also asked to specify the length of time they had worked with computers. This ranged from a minimum of 6 days to a maximum of 10 years.

It was noted that the students' previous experiences in the use of computers were very mixed ranging from total ignorance (57.9%) to considerable experience. This mix continues throughout training and has implications for future course structures.

With regard to the students' experience with computers in the clinical areas, less than half of them (45.4%) had encountered the use of computers during their practice placements; this involved computerised nurse information systems and patient administration systems. Of those who had such experience, 62.7% commented on the extent of their involvement with the computers. It was disappointing to see that only 3.9% of the students were allowed to use the computers on the wards and this involvement was reported as minimal.

IT systems are only as good as the people who use them. As nurses are being used as a resource to capture or produce data, it is essential that they learn to give clear, concise and accurate information and to understand its purpose and its contribution to patient care. The nurse's role must not be limited to that of data gatherer or data processor. It is therefore important for students to see computing skills as useful and relevant to their everyday work. They must be oriented to information systems in the clinical setting, to view the system in use and ask questions about its functions in order to gain a good insight into the working of the system. However, the study found little or no evidence of encouragement for students to use their clinical placements in this way. This would seem to be another example of poor integration between theory and practice.

With the traditional system of training followed by the students in the sample, the majority of learning takes place on the ward and it is here that future attitudes to the use of technology will be established. It is therefore important that every opportunity is taken to capitalise on the presence of ward-based information systems within the educational process.

Students will only see the usefulness of computing skills if the technology is available on the wards and it is found to be relevant and useful in practice; while the technology is not available for use, the remaining 54.6% will continue to have little understanding of the management use of computers.

Respondents were also asked about their use of computers for work and recreation. Only 25% of the respondents had access to a computer at their present accommodation or residence. For those who did use a computer, it was mainly utilised for games and/or word processing. In exploring the personal use of computers for specified activities, the findings showed that the personal use of the computer as an educational or personal tool was poor (Table 11.2). It was particularly surprising to note the limited use of word processing, although this is a very useful tool for students. When asked about their use of computers in education, the most popular responses were CAL, games and word processing (Table 11.3). Even then the number of students using the computers for these activities was small.

Table 11.2 Personal use of the computer ($n = 183$)
Do you personally use the computer for:

	Yes	No	No response
Word processing	48 (26.2%)	95 (51.9%)	40 (21.9%)
Data collection	25 (13.7%)	101 (52.2%)	57 (31.1%)
Spreadsheets	8 (4.4%)	109 (59.6%)	66 (36.1%)
Problem solving	15 (8.2%)	107 (58.5%)	61 (33.3%)
CAL	46 (25.1%)	84 (45.9%)	53 (29%)
Desktop publishing	6 (3.3%)	110 (60.1%)	67 (36.6%)
Games	67 (36.6%)	71 (38.8%)	45 (24.6%)

Table 11.3 Use of school computers ($n = 171$)
What do you use the school computers for?

Data management	13 (7.6%)
Word processing	28 (16.3%)
CAL	70 (41.0%)
Problem solving	26 (15.2%)
Games	34 (19.9%)

Knowledge of facilities available

76.5% of the respondents knew that there was a computer laboratory or room within their School of Nursing, although in two schools the knowledge of this facility was poor. However, the computers in the Schools of Nursing appeared to be underused. 49.2% of the respondents said that they rarely used the computers and 48.1% did not use the computers at all. This would not appear to be effective use of resources. Why are students not using computers? 83% of the respondents offered explanations. The main reasons given (Table 11.4) for the low use of computers were:

- lack of confidence and knowledge to use the computers
- lack of encouragement and support on the part of nurse educators
- location of computers was not easily accessible
- lack of time
- lack of knowledge about the availability of the facilities.

When respondents were asked about their access to computers, there was a great disparity of opinions expressed. There also appeared to be considerable confusion over what was available. This area warrants further investigation. However, it reflects an unsatisfactory state of affairs and suggests a lack of awareness of the schools' policies governing student access to computers intended for their use. It may also indicate failure on the part of the Schools of Nursing in making the policy known and also a lack of explicit policies for IT within the curriculum. Student use of IT can only become a reality if the technology is available. Policies governing access to computers should be made known and time made available for the students to use the computers. It could be argued that students should be sufficiently motivated to gain access for themselves, in the spirit of self-directed learning. However, they may be easily discouraged by lack of support, poor access and lack of time. Computers can be very frustrating and negative attitudes are easily engendered.

Table 11.4 Reasons for low use of school computers ($n = 61$)

Lack of confidence and knowledge	18 (29.5%)
No encouragement and poor support	13 (21.3%)
Location—not easily accessible	10 (16.4%)
Lack of time	10 (16.4%)
No knowledge of the facilities	10 (16.4%)

Formal educational opportunities

The survey findings suggested that students are not being adequately prepared for the many issues that they are likely to face in their professional role in an IT environment.

Only 34.4% of the respondents are currently being taught computing in their Schools of Nursing and this is largely limited to educational and personal use. The time allocated for this teaching is not uniform. In one School of Nursing, the students were given a computer familiarity course incorporating keyboard and word processing skills during their introductory course and at the end of their second year of training, whilst in the other Schools a basic introduction to computers and keyboard skills was given. The time allocated varied from a couple of sessions during introductory course only, or during the students' first and second modules. For one School, computer training was arranged on a scheduled basis on the students' first wards of training when they received a 3-hour session. No formal teaching programme was indicated in two Schools of Nursing.

Some Schools of Nursing are making attempts to increase the students' awareness of IT but the preparation of the student continues without a recognition on the part of nurse educators of many of the important issues which relate to the use of IT.

The responses received regarding the students' understanding of the terms such as 'resource management', 'resource management initiatives' and 'hospital information support systems' (Table 11.5) suggests a poor knowledge of these issues. 95.6% of the respondents indicated that the resource management initiatives were not discussed (Table 11.6). Nurses need to be aware of current issues such as these, which will have a significant effect on their professional practice. However, the survey suggests that students are largely unaware of the information initiatives currently being introduced into the NHS and the changes which nurses will face with the introduction of IT. This reinforces the point that nurse educators are neither taking the initiative nor encouraging the students to examine these issues.

Even in those Schools of Nursing where the importance of understanding IT is recognised, learning experiences appear to be confined to teaching students to operate computers as an educational or personal tool, mainly involving CAL or word processing activities (Table 11.3).

Table 11.5 Understanding of terms (n = 183)

Do you know the meaning of the following terms?

	Yes	No	No response
Resource management	56 (30.6%)	126 (68.9%)	1 (0.5%)
Resource management initiatives	20 (10.9%)	159 (86.9%)	4 (2.2%)
Hospital information support systems	30 (16.4%)	150 (82%)	3 (1.6%)

Table 11.6 Respondents' perception of discussion of specific topics within the curriculum (n = 183)

	Yes	No	No response
The resource management initiatives	7 (3.8%)	175 (95.6%)	1 (0.5%)
Use of computers within the NHS	53 (29%)	130 (71%)	0
Systems design concepts	4 (2.2%)	179 (97.8%)	0
System evaluation and selection	5 (2.7%)	178 (97.3%)	0
Data versus information (data collection and coding)	13 (7.1%)	170 (92.9%)	0
Methods of data entry	22 (12%)	160 (87.4%)	1 (0.5%)
Use of information for decision making in hospital	28 (15.3%)	154 (84.2%)	1 (0.5%)
Data security (destruction, accidental access and loss)	31 (16.9%)	150 (82%)	2 (1.1%)
The Data Protection Act	41 (22.4%)	142 (77.6%)	0

Cobin (1983) and Eaton (1987) both suggest that CAL prompts general thinking and problem-solving skills, as well as helping with the acquisition of basic computing skills. Although these activities do provide a valuable introduction to IT, only teaching such skills by themselves restricts the students' experience to a narrow aspect of information technology. Skills training alone will not prepare students for the many issues that they are likely to encounter in their role as professional nurses.

It has already been argued that the profession needs nurses who are proactive in their attitude to computers if they are to have any measure of control over how IT will affect their work. This requires an understanding of IT and its relevance in health care, including ethical, legal, social and political issues. Nurses must be knowledgeable about computer functions, specification design and the use of technology in their own field, and to be able to project future uses.

Unfortunately the responses from the study suggest that the necessary educational opportunities have not been available. The majority of respondents indicated that topics such as those shown in Table 11.6 were not discussed during their course of study, although an understanding of these topics is essential for the successful use of computer systems. It is also of concern that the nature and extent of IT experience varied considerably between different schools.

Dowling (1980) pointed out that the ineffective facilitation of change can also result in 'computerphobia'. Comments received from a small minority of the study sample indicated that some resistance and computerphobia may have been present. For example:

'Did not come into nursing to waste time with computers.'

'I don't like them, they are impersonal.'

'I am already turned off by the whole concept of computers.'

'I found computers make me very ill physically. The VDU screens regularly gave me eye strain and stomach aches.'

'They confuse me and they frighten me because of the possible effects if they went wrong and shut down.'

Organisation and teaching of IT

Only two of the seven Schools of Nursing had an identified nurse teacher with a degree of expertise to deal with the organisation and teaching of IT. The role of these teachers can be crucial in the promotion of effective use of computers. The two Schools with an identified teacher appeared from the results to be the most innovative schools in the study. In the Schools where there were no designated teachers for this role, student involvement in information technology was limited or non-existent. Lack of support and encouragement to use IT in these schools was also expressed by the study sample.

Attitudes of students

The findings revealed that the majority of respondents (83%) had a positive attitude towards the use of computers for nursing and that some respondents appeared to recognise the role of computers. This is reflected in their comments. 71% of the respondents strongly wanted to have some input or choice in the decision-making process of designing computer systems for nurses' use. This suggests some grounds for optimism regarding future practitioners' attitudes to IT and their motivation to learn and participate in aspects concerning IT in nursing.

Students' expressed needs

The results of the survey suggest that respondents perceived themselves as having a low level of knowledge about computers and IT; by contrast respondents expressed a desire for a high level of knowledge. 79.8% of the students would have liked to have been taught if a course had been available.

Respondents were asked to make suggestions as to what should be done to meet their present and future needs. 59.6% of the students responded to this open question. It is not clear whether those who did not respond were unable to by virtue of their lack of knowledge, or for some other reason. However, the comments that were received were voluminous, and a variety of needs were expressed. The most common need expressed was for basic teaching of IT to be provided during their training (47.7%). One respondent wrote a paragraph emphasising the need for education.

20.5% of the respondents wanted more information about the relevance of computers to nursing and the issues surrounding the use of computers in nursing. For example one respondent made this comment: 'I would like to know the Health Authority's policy on computer-held information and on computer use.' This comment suggests a concern with data security and confidentiality, but a majority (82%) of the students had previously stated that the issues of data security and the Data Protection Act were not discussed with them during their course of study (Table 11.6).

Effective computer use requires extra time for 'hands-on' experience if students are to become confident. Independent learning was pointed out by Lange (1988) as a very important factor to encourage computer use, so it was not surprising that this need was expressed by 17.8% of the students, together with a need for more regular training (14%). The comments suggested that the computer training provided by the Schools of Nursing was not uniform and occurred on a sporadic basis. Skiba (1985) has emphasised that IT education and training must be a consistent thread woven throughout the curriculum. Otherwise, the skills gained are soon lost. It is important that training is structured if students are to make full use of IT, commencing in introductory course, reinforced at regular intervals and followed up with continuing education after qualification so as to provide a continuum of learning experience.

Implications for nurse education

The results of the study showed that the students' current level of knowledge of IT was poor. Therefore, despite the positive attitude held towards the use of computers for nursing, because of their lack of knowledge, utilisation of the computers as an educational or personal tool was difficult, resulting in the resource being underused. At the same time the wider applications of the computer as a management tool could not be considered. The need for education and training in IT has been established.

Nurse education has been shown to be lagging behind despite the expressed concerns to provide nurses with computer literacy skills (Andreoli & Musser 1985, Eaton 1987, Peel 1990, Sultana 1990). The results of the survey suggest that within most Welsh Schools of Nursing there was little evidence of a proactive approach to education in IT. The introduction of IT was in many instances uncoordinated and in some instances no integration of IT education within the curriculum was evident. Students' exposure to and use of computers during basic nurse education continues to be sporadic. Fundamental management issues relating to the use of IT were not well covered, so it must be assumed that students are inadequately prepared to cope with the professional implications of using IT in health care.

A factor identified by the study as inhibiting the utilisation of computers was the lack of encouragement and support on the part of nurse educators. This seems to suggest that nurse educators are themselves in the uninitiate stage (Hassett 1984) and that this is having a direct effect on students. Fundamental changes in the role and behaviour of both nurse educators and senior managers are required.

If nurses are to adopt a more dynamic approach within an IT environment, they must be adequately prepared. However, the results from this study suggest that students will not be at the 'informed user' level when they qualify, given the current incoherent education in IT and the expectation that nurses in the future will be able to use the computer as today they use the telephone will not be met. The present system of training has passively impeded the development of computer literacy and familiarity with the concepts and objectives associated with IT and nurse educators must recognise the problems of the present system. IT education can no longer be omitted as a subject from any nursing curriculum. There should be provision for IT at different levels, that is at an 'informed user' level,'proficient user' level and at an advanced level for those who would wish to be developers of computer systems. Only then can nurses successfully cope with and shape the changes in nursing that IT will bring.

CONCLUSIONS AND RECOMMENDATIONS

Our future nurses must be computer literate, i.e. the nurse must have knowledge about the computer, be able to learn by using the computer and be able to use the computer as an effective tool in the nursing profession. Nurse educators must adjust curricula to include discussions on the limitations, social, legal and ethical issues of the use of computers in nursing. This must also allow for hands-on skills where the students will be encouraged to use CAL programs for part of the course as an educational tool, use word processing as a personal tool, use library search and statistical programs as part of education in research methods and a hospital information support system as part of clinical experience.

Further developments at an advanced level to enable nurses to become proficient users and developers of computer systems must also be considered by providing continuing computer education at different levels of post-registration education. This could follow the guidelines suggested by Ronald & Skiba (1987).

Some changes in the existing curriculum will be required for the successful integration of IT education into the nursing curriculum. Participation by nurse educators in a common project focusing on the development of a framework for IT education must be encouraged. All four National Boards have given some attention to the problem in recent years, but the United Kingdom Central Council (UKCC) is the body responsible for determining the standard, kind and content of professional education, and they must give a clear lead in this area.

Integration of the use of computers as a tool throughout the nursing curriculum can only be successful if it is planned, supported, and above all resourced. Appropriate hardware, software and support material and personnel must be available. This has been difficult in the past because computer equipment has been relatively expensive and has had a low priority in the competition for funding. Prices have fallen, but the funding issue remains important, particularly as the responsibility for funds is removed from the National Boards to be administered within the contracting arrangements which have followed the reforms of the NHS.

To blend the use of computer technology into the practice of nursing and at the same time maintain quality care, basic knowledge and IT skills should be a requirement of all nurse educators. Education managers should initiate change and provide a climate in which the desired change can take place by ensuring that teachers attend IT workshops or courses inside as well as outside the NHS, thereby increasing levels of knowledge and skills in this area. Until nurse educators gain the necessary skills it may be necessary to employ computer educators or IT specialists.

REFERENCES

Anderson J, Grémy F, Pages J C 1974 Education in informatics of health personnel. North-Holland/Elsevier, Amsterdam

Andreoli K, Musser L A 1985 Computers in nursing care: the state of the art. Nursing Outlook 33(1): 16–21

Chapman C 1974 Nursing education curriculum content. Queen's Nursing Journal 17(7): 149–152

Cobin J 1983 Combining computers with caring. Nursing Times 79(41): 24–26

Cox H C, Harsanyi B, Dean L C 1987 Computers and nursing: application to practice, education and research. Appleton & Lange, Norwalk, USA

Department of Health and Social Security 1983 The NHS Management Inquiry Report (The Griffith's Report). HMSO, London

Department of Health and Social Security (1984) Steering Group on Health Services Information: a further report on the collection and use of information about hospital clinical activity in the National Health Service (Korner Report). HMSO, London

Dowling A 1980 Do hospital staff interfere with computer system implementation? Health Care Management Review 5(4): 23–32

Eaton N 1987 Teaching computing to nursing students. Senior Nurse 7(3): 28–29

Fardell J 1989 Fighting together. Nursing Times 85(11): 31–32

Freeman R 1990 Minister launches IT strategy. The British Journal of Healthcare Computing 7(1): 9

Hassett M R 1984 Computers and nursing education in the 1980s. Nursing Outlook 32(1): 34–36

HMSO 1984 The Data Protection Act 1984. HMSO, London

HMSO 1989a A Government White Paper: Working for patients. HMSO, London

HMSO 1989b A strategy for nursing. Report of seminar organised by Department of Health and Social Security Nursing Division, October 1989

Jarvis J 1988 Computers and managing nursing. Senior Nurse 7(3): 25–26

Lange L L 1988 Computer anxiety, computer skills, computer use and interest in learning about computers before and after a computer literacy course. In: Lochlas T (ed) Nursing and computers. Third international symposium on nursing use of computers and information science, Dublin. C V Mosby, St Louis, pp 205–215

Massie S 1989 Health carers: Technologists or technocrats. Senior Nurse 9(5): 7–8

Melia K 1990 Computer ethics. Nursing Times 85(29): 62–63

Merrison A 1979 Report of the Royal Commission on the NHS. HMSO, London

Newbern V B 1985 Computer literacy in nursing education. Nursing Clinics of North America 20(3): 549–556

Peel V 1990 Dual approach needed to tackle low IT skills. The Health Service Journal 100(5219): 1377

Ronald J S, Skiba D J 1987 Guidelines for basic computer education in nursing. National League For Nursing, New York

Schwirinan P 1983 Editorial: The future is ours if.... Computers in Nursing 1(3): 1

Skiba D J 1985 Interactive computer experiences. Nursing Clinics of North America 20(3): 577–583

Sultana N 1990 Nurses' attitudes towards computerisation in clinical practice. Journal of Advanced Nursing 15(6): 696–702

12

Ethical implications of nursing informatics

P. Wainwright

Introduction	Is technology neutral?
The moral nature of nursing	The appeal of technology
The place of nursing informatics	and unitary concepts of health
Ethics and informatics	Conclusions
In search of efficiency	

INTRODUCTION

The fields of nursing informatics and ethics both cover considerable ground: to attempt a consideration of the one from the perspective of the other is a massive undertaking. This chapter will therefore necessarily be partial and selective, focusing on a limited selection of the many possible issues and raising questions about nursing informatics which seem to me to be about moral issues.

THE MORAL NATURE OF NURSING

There is an extensive body of literature concerning the moral nature of nursing, and I do not propose to enter into a lengthy review of it here. However, I will summarise briefly some of the key concepts. Moral philosophy is in essence about what is good, and in particular what will lead to good or well being for individuals and people in general. Nursing is concerned with the well being of patients or clients and about ways of seeking and fostering their best interests. If we accept that nursing is about a concern for individuals and their needs, rather than just the skilled execution of certain technical tasks, then nursing is a moral activity, and any consideration of nursing must include an account of the ethics of nursing: theories of nursing must include ethical theory.

Central to an understanding of nursing is the notion of caring, and again more has been written already about caring than I can hope to cover here. Writers such as Benner (1984), Noddings (1986) and Watson (1985) in particular have discussed the nature of care and caring from an ethical and a nursing perspective.

Many writers have also discussed other moral qualities required of or exhibited by the nurse, suggesting virtues such as honesty, compassion, benevolence, courage, and conscientiousness. Nursing is what MacIntyre has called a 'practice', an activity characterised in part by virtue, and the relationship between the nurse and the patient is a fiduciary one, based on trust (MacIntyre 1985).

Because of its moral nature, nursing is about much more than the performance of tasks, however technically demanding they might be. Nursing is a discretionary activity, requiring professional judgement, and there are many situations in nursing in which there is no right answer, many problems for which there are no solutions. Above all, nursing is about the relationship between the nurse and the patient, a relationship between two human beings.

THE PLACE OF NURSING INFORMATICS

For all of the above reasons the nurse is morally obliged to seek to develop and improve her knowledge and skills, in the pursuit of excellence in her practice. This is one of the characteristic features of 'practice' in the sense in which MacIntyre uses the word and is clearly essential if nurses are to justify the trust placed in them by patients and if they are to pursue the patients' best interests as if they were their own.

This striving for excellence requires that practitioners are willing to adopt new methods and techniques in any area of their practice, in so far as these new methods can be shown to be beneficial. Information handling is one of the most crucial of nursing activities, so clearly a science which is dedicated to improving our ability to collect and process data, to transform and use it effectively, must be a strong contender for time in the nursing curriculum.

However, in allocating time and other resources to informatics we must keep in mind the need to justify the investment in terms of the likely benefits. This concern is born out in the informatics literature. For example, Redmond (1983), in a review of the development of computing in the NHS, describes plans introduced in 1967 for research and development to support projects with three main objectives:

- to ensure better patient care
- to increase clinical and administrative efficiency
- to improve management and research facilities.

An editorial in Information Technology in Nursing (Anon 1989) throws out the challenge to 'demonstrate ... how computers can improve the care that I give', and Taylor & Cameron (1990) refer to the principle objective of the Resource Management Initiative of 1986 as being the introduction of a new approach to managing resources which results in measurable improvements in patient care. As sub-objectives clinicians were to be provided with information which enabled them to:

- identify areas of waste and inefficiency
- benefit from clinical group discussion and review
- highlight areas which could most benefit from more resources
- identify and expose the health care consequences of given financial policies and constraints
- understand the comparative costs of future health care options and hold informed debates about such costs.

There is thus a strong moral drive behind the development of health care informatics in that it is justified on the grounds of improvements in care. It is perhaps unfortunate that a recent report from the Brunel University team evaluating the six pilot sites for Resource Management in the UK found that they 'have failed to measurably improve patient care' and that 'RM cannot yet be said to have produced a way of working that has demonstrated its ability to achieve significant measurable patient benefits' (Anon 1991). The pilot sites had at the time of reporting consumed £10 million, and the English Department of Health (DOH) budget for RM for 1991–1992 was in excess of £90 million.

It would be unfair to lay the blame for the apparent failure of RM entirely at the door of informatics, but distributive justice is a key concern in health care ethics and examples of this kind highlight the need to look critically at the investment of large sums of money in technology. It would not seem unreasonable to expect such investment to produce improvements in care. However, given that there will always be competing demands for any money, the debate about the best way to spend money will always have a moral component.

ETHICS AND INFORMATICS

A review of the literature suggests that there is a paucity of publications which discuss what I will call, for convenience, the ethics of informatics. There does not seem to be the same kind of ethical debate about informatics as there is about, for example, euthanasia, human fertility or abortion. However, if we take the usual kind of definition of nursing informatics, that it is the 'combination of computer science, information science and nursing science designed to assist in the management and processing of nursing data, information and knowledge to support the practice of nursing and the delivery of care' (Graves & Corcoran 1989), it would seem that we are confronted by ethical issues at every turn, and that it cannot be sufficient to argue that informatics just develops the techniques in some kind of amoral, value free way.

For example, it seems to me that information has no independent existence. Information always relates to something or someone, and the ethical importance of the information is in direct proportion to the ethical importance of that which it represents. In manipulating the information we are to some extent manipulating the subject of that information.

Some authors do tackle ethical questions, but these tend to be concerned with issues such as privacy and confidentiality. Nurses have been concerned about confidentiality from the very beginning of the development of the profession, and Plant (1983), in a discussion of confidentiality and data protection, quotes from Florence Nightingale's Notes on Nursing. Miss Nightingale wrote 'and remember every nurse should be one who is to be depended upon, in other words, capable of being a "confidential" nurse ... she must be no gossip, no vain talker, she should never answer questions about her sick except to those who have a right to ask them'.

As with so much else that Florence Nightingale wrote, these sentiments are still valid and could form the basis for any discussion of confidentiality, privacy and data protection.

Walsh & Cortez (1991), discussing the application of computerised data systems in quality assurance (QA) programs, acknowledge that clinical systems pay considerable attention to confidentiality and security, but make the point that QA applications, by linking individual patient data with practice and performance data, greatly broaden the area of confidentiality and liability.

This is a good example of the way in which linked computer systems bring together data in ways in which subjects may know nothing about, creating new information about them. Walsh & Cortez do not have much to say about the ethical implications of such information generation, but they do make some recommendations for security, such as locking terminals when not in use, restricting access to those authorised to use the system, maintaining proper password controls and so on.

In a similar vein, a speaker at a seminar on primary care (Bradley, cited by Warren 1991) said that 'General Practitioners have the richest access to data ... of immense value to organizations concerned with the provision, planning and effective management of health care services'. The same speaker acknowledged that no work has been done yet on addressing patient consent in this respect, although the European Community may introduce legislation in the future, and that 'the value of a greater understanding of society and the value of allowing an individual to keep information about himself and his life private may be contradictory'.

Another speaker at the same seminar (Robinson, cited by Warren 1991), emphasising the role of the new referral letter as a major source of information for planners, argued that the loss of individual freedom which results from the use of such information in ways other than that for which it was obtained, when set against the gains to the community, is a sacrifice that patients and GPs ought to be prepared to make.

On a cautionary note, Jackson (cited in Brown & Warren 1991) warns us that while computers speed up data handling, they make it possible to get the wrong answer faster.

All of this presents the nurse with a real dilemma. Typically it is nurses who gather much patient data, and indeed the quantity of information collected through some approaches to the nursing process has led some people to be critical of the process of nursing assessment. However, when the nurse interviewed the patient and wrote the answers down in the Kardex she or he could give the patient some explanation as to why the questions were being asked, what would happen to the information, and who else might see it. When nurses enter data into hospital information systems they lose control over it and no longer have any means of knowing who may use it and for what purpose. It is unlikely that patients ever give informed consent for the disclosure of personal information in this way.

The teaching of informatics is one area where a consideration of ethical issues might be expected. It is therefore interesting to consider the work of Bryson (1991) on the teaching of computer literacy. Bryson describes research intended to develop subsets of instructional objectives, based on the Minnesota Educational

Consortium's seven domains of computer literacy, and to ask educators to rate these objectives for importance within the curriculum.

The seven domains of computer literacy defined by the Minnesota Consortium are:

- programming and algorithm skills
- skills in computer usage
- hardware and software principles
- major uses and application principles
- limitations of computers
- personal and social aspects
- relevant values and attitudes.

From these Bryson developed 74 sub-objectives, and of these it would appear that six were in some way related to ethical concepts. Five of these were in Domain 6, Personal and Social aspects:

- know the importance of confidentiality of computerised medical information and records
- know about the laws regarding computer information
- be concerned about what data is collected and how the data is used
- be concerned about the dehumanisation of patient care resulting from the use of the computer
- know that the use of Hospital Information System may result in a power shift within the hospital organisation; the computer centre can control who has access to information

and one was in Domain 7, Relevant Values and Attitudes:

- know about ethical/legal issues and concerns relating to information processing in health care.

However, most of these are associated more with issues of privacy and confidentiality, rather than with broader moral issues. In general it seems as though it is taken for granted that the development of informatics is beneficial and desirable, and that all we need to do is take a few simple precautions with regard to security. There is a great deal of question begging, and not much analysis of moral issues. This problem is typified by Squire's (1983) advice that 'to quote from a well known medical guideline, "never do harm"'. He goes on to suggest what amounts to a code of conduct:

- we should not harm the service we provide by introducing untested systems which destroy the confidence of managers in the use of the technology

- we should avoid the introduction of expensive systems until we can be sure that they can meet the needs of the service not only locally but in a way that allows inter-changeability and computer to computer communication
- we must ensure that our systems are secure and that the information stored within them is only used for legitimate purposes controlled by an agreed ethical policy
- we should not destroy the credibility of the technology by introducing systems that create additional work or produce irrelevant information through it being either inaccurate or time-expired.

IN SEARCH OF EFFICIENCY

History provides a fascinating parallel with today's concerns about the efficient use of resources. Reverby (1987), in her study of American nursing between 1850 and 1945, describes the increasing interest shown at the beginning of the 20th century by the profession in scientific management and efficiency. According to Reverby, the ambiguity of terms such as 'efficiency' and 'scientific management' gave them a wide appeal to nurse leaders.

Nurse educators were anxious to include more basic science and more objective study of methods and practices, and while hospital administrators saw efficiency as a way of getting more work from the workforce, nurse leaders had a language they could use to demand more science in the curriculum or the hiring of aids to do more mundane work. The idea that efficiency schemes could improve care and free nursing from drudgery was attractive, and the methods of efficiency engineers were seen as the means to produce scientific, objective evidence of the need to upgrade nursing.

As Reverby suggests, it was ironic that the methods that had made industrial work more mechanical were seen by nurses as the means to escape from 'martinet discipline, routinism, and institutionalism'. A nurse writing on hospital economics claimed that 'scientific management of tasks improves the spirit of workers', while the introduction of standardisation techniques and time and motion studies would make it possible to restore dignity to nursing and rekindle its ideals.

Before long nurses began to fear that the new techniques of management would make nursing into something that contradicted its greatest ideals. There were accusations that efficiency approaches led to the mechanisation of the human soul, that they would take the heart out of nursing, and leave the nurse without an individual identity and sense of responsibility. The approach to the hospital as an industrial plant left the student nurse with little knowledge of any patient as a whole, while the concentration on task analysis and division of labour led to the development of the 'functional' method of nursing. Of this, one nursing educator noted:

> The patient is not the unit or centre of thought. But the work to be done is classified into: beds to be made, baths to be given, temperatures to be taken, treatments to be given, diets to be prepared and served, medications to be given, charting to be done, dressings to be done etc. The thing to be done is the unit and centre of thought and endeavour.

Taylor & Cameron (1990) argue that the most important element required from nursing management systems is the cost of the patient's nursing care; this must be as accurate as possible and be 'related to the diagnosis of each ... patient'. The only way to obtain accurate costs is 'to break down nursing activities into some detail and to record what nurses actually do'. Nursing activities can then be given a standard cost which becomes 'a fixed price to the clinician'. Nurses must be prepared to categorise patients into groups and engage in 'discussions of a standard profile of care for each one of these ... groups'. Jones & Buchanan (1989) say that 'activity monitoring has become one of the standard ways of providing a representation or definition of ward-based work.'

IS TECHNOLOGY NEUTRAL?

Supporters of informatics and the use of technology in nursing appear to be guilty of question begging on a grand scale. As Chandler (1990) suggests, for those who believe technology is neutral the only legitimate criticism is of the use that is made of it. However, Chandler goes on to argue that this presupposes that the technology does not embody priorities which may run contrary to our purpose or subvert our values, and that it allows us to choose how we use it. According to Chandler, computers can never be general-purpose, content-free tools and using a computer can transform one's intentions according to an inexplicit but unavoidable ideology.

The problem, according to Chandler, is that the computer denies the human origin of information. We refer to information handling and information technology, but Chandler insists there is no information in computers, only data. Human beings create information by interpreting the evidence of their senses and through negotiating with other human beings. In a human community interpretations are multifarious, so no one interpretation can be absolute: meaning is negotiated through human discourse. When we detach the knowers from the known we divorce knowledge from the community, from history, from wisdom. The language of the computer culture threatens to redefine the world in its own terms.

Chandler also points out another dimension of the reductionism of data handling systems: the importance accorded to data is magnified by storage in large quantities and acquires spurious authority. Every time data is stored on computers the value attached to other sources of information is diminished.

Ford (1990) has suggested that the full impact of computer use and the implications for nursing have yet to be understood. He differentiates between Utopian ideologies, which hold that the use of the computer in itself is neutral, and Romantic ideologies which hold that far from being neutral, machines have a negative effect, that they are essentially dehumanising and that they alienate man from nature. Ford also quotes Ihde, who suggests that while technology is not neutral, its effects may be either positive or negative and that there can be a symbiotic relationship with them; he also quotes Burch, who thinks that technology transforms experience, for better or worse, 'and ultimately shapes human thinking and being'.

The notion that the use of technology shapes human thinking is interesting, and of some significance for nurses. Many authors have described the development of expert systems, decision support systems, and computerised patient care documentation for nursing. By definition, these systems rely on the ability to standardise, and to develop rules that have wide application. Some of these are built around standardised nursing diagnoses (for example, Strength & Keen-Payne 1991) while others develop rules from existing practices and records of past problems and their solutions (Jones 1991). However, the development and use of such systems may result in the adoption of certain modes of thought or approaches to problem solving which may run counter to current ideas about professional practice and the nature of expertise.

Sinclair (1990) suggests that the computer can change the definition of expertise. As the quantity of information expands to exceed the capacity of the human brain the characteristics of computer memory can make lack of factual knowledge less important. However, Sinclair quotes Bereiter and Scardamalia, who argue that true expertise requires the absorption of large amounts of knowledge to form complex knowledge structures. Experts perceive problems differently from novices, 'creatively generating abstract principles from particular problems which may then be utilised to address future problems'.

Benner & Wrubel (1989) stress the experiential element in the development of expertise, and both they and Bereiter and Scardamalia discuss the expert's intuitive ability to perceive problems holistically and rapidly to single out relevant information, while Sinclair argues that expert systems cannot mimic important aspects of human intelligence such as judgement and intuition. Computers attempt to simulate logical thinking by making inferences from lists of rules, but intuitive expertise is not reducible to rules.

The debate about the place of expert systems and nursing diagnoses looks likely to continue for some time yet. On a more mundane level, however, the use of computers and information systems may have more immediate effects. For example, Ford (1990) suggests that while computers can relieve nurses of clerical and monitoring tasks, decrease errors and increase time for patients,'the elimination of manual recording of patient variables may have the adverse effect of reducing the nurse's clinical awareness' and 'it is likely that nursing observations and notes may not lend themselves to being automated without compromising the quality of such notes'. The use of computers may decrease the nurse's sensitivity to the patient's situation, with the risk of reducing the patient to a distant object, with implications for the helping relationship.

Ford further suggests that the use of computers in care settings may detract from the development of a trusting relationship between nurse and patient. This is because the computer may take up nursing time which would otherwise have been spent with the patient, thus reducing opportunities for developing trust, and because computers are associated by some people with the misuse of information, computer crime and so on, and this may provoke mistrust on the part of the patient and his/her family. People may feel that the computer is in control, and this in turn may foster passivity and dependence, while the production of printed care plans and notes may encourage a sense of depersonalisation. Finally Ford notes that computers are biased towards rational-analytic thinking styles rather than the non-rational/creative approach. Computer use may thus favour rational thinking rather than creative thinking, with a tendency to limit thinking and narrow nurses' perspective.

THE APPEAL OF TECHNOLOGY AND UNITARY CONCEPTS OF HEALTH

In an earlier section of this chapter I raised the question of the contribution of informatics to improvements in patient care. But what constitutes good, or better, care is in many ways a moral question. Health policy makers and planners have written a great deal of late about the concept of 'health gain' as the objective of health care, and advances in technology, including information technology, have been hailed as among the most important contributing factors in achieving health gain in the future.

In a detailed discussion of the notion of health gain, Evans et al (1991) argue that the notion of 'health' which underpins the appeal to technology is essentially one which is mechanistic and reductionist, an account of health in terms of nominal function and physiological or biochemical measurement,'rather than understanding these indicators in the light of the patient's experience'. Such an approach to health care reflects a positivistic system, regarded as free from values and therefore neutral. The reductionist and positivistic approach is also unitary—that is, health is perceived as being the same wherever and whenever you look and health status is portrayed as a single point on the same continuum for all.

'Health gain' is taken to mean 'improvements in health status', and may relate to individuals or groups. However, health gain in a group or population may not equate to health gain for any one individual, and vice versa. Measures which may statistically improve the health of the group may detract from the well being of an individual, whether through an idiosyncratic reaction to (for example) fluoride in the water supply or routine vaccination, or because of an individual's idiosyncratic view of health and well being, as with users of tobacco, alcohol or other mind-altering substances.

There is much discussion of the importance of patient outcomes, the assumption being that health gain can be measured in terms of outcomes which lead to the twin objectives of 'adding years to life and life to years'. As Evans et al point out, the former is at least measurable, even though its desirability may be disputed. (Some years ago a cartoon appeared in one of the journals, showing two patients in the day room of the geriatric ward. One was saying to the other, 'Just think, if we hadn't stopped smoking we would have missed all this!')

There is much more dispute about what constitutes 'added life'. Evans et al suggest that improved mobility, for example, may be greatly valued by one person, but totally irrelevant to another, even though both have the same degree of handicap. Society is characterised by the diversity of values and goals 'which variously enrich the lives of different patients'. A commitment to 'added life' is therefore open ended: there is no limit to the kinds of things patients may demand. What counts as 'better or more desirable' life is the subject of moral debate, and many of the goals identified by health professionals as desirable for their patients 'appeal to a familiar but not a universal conception of a good and enriched life'. To specify what is meant by 'added life' is to make 'an explicitly moral judgement'.

By the same token, outcome measurement is at least controversial and, according to Evans et al, there are 'questions concerning its very coherence'. They cite as an example the treatment of mild hypertension. This is a medical problem, and the desired outcome would be a return to a normal measurement, which could be achieved with hypotensive medication. The patient may be asymptomatic, but both he and his wife could suffer from the side-effects (lethargy, irritability, impotence) of the medication. Whether there has been a successful outcome depends on your point of view. Evans et al do not discuss it, but there is also the concept of a 'good death' to further complicate matters.

These latter examples illustrate the difficulty of reducing notions of improved well being, and the recognition of the patient as an individual, to the level of simple physiological measurement. However, nursing theorists have long argued that individualised care leading to improvements in well being is precisely what nursing sets out to achieve. The importance of sensitivity to the individual is discussed by Noddings (1986), who argues that caring involves adopting the other person's frame of reference in order to see things from his or her point of view. To care, says Noddings, is to act 'not by fixed rule but by affection and regard'. This means that it is likely that the actions of the carer will be varied, rather than rule-bound: 'her actions, while predictable in a global sense, will be unpredictable in detail. Variation is to be expected if the one claiming to care really cares, for her engrossment is in the variable and never fully understood other, in the particular other, in a particular set of circumstances.'

Noddings' arguments would suggest that not only will a caring nurse respond in different ways to different patients who have the same medical condition, but also that different nurses may quite reasonably act in different ways with any one patient, as they bring their own understanding and concern to the situation.

CONCLUSIONS

I think it is clear that any study of informatics must include a consideration of moral or ethical implications. To the extent that informatics can lead to a better understanding of the processes of information management, or to more efficient or effective care, or faster or more accurate diagnosis, the subject has considerable potential as a force for moral good. Informatics may also have an important place in the professional curriculum, providing powerful tools and models for learning and for simulation and safe experimentation.

On the other hand, I have tried to show that there are potential dangers, especially if one is caught up with enthusiasm for a new subject, or one falls victim to a naïve belief in the ability, indeed the superior ability, of technology to solve all problems. It is important to remember that there are other considerations to take into account, and an instrumental, reductionist, technological approach may deny many of the essentially human characteristics of care and caring, and of professional work. Peter Verduin and Paul Epping have more to say about this elsewhere in this book.

Above all, I would stress the need for consideration of the ethical issues within any enterprise involving informatics and information technology. It is often said that one of the key questions concerning the morality of a course of action is the underlying intention, but the end does not necessarily justify the means. There is always the risk that we will change our behaviour in order to support the information systems and to meet their needs, rather than ensuring that the application of informatics meets the needs of patients and supports the advance of patient-centred care. What amounts to good patient care is inescapably a moral question; the extent to which informatics and information technology improve the care of patients can only be answered if, along with the technical issues, the ethical issues are given equal weight.

REFERENCES

Anon 1989 Editorial. Information Technology in Nursing 1(2): 19

Anon 1991 Research reveals failings of resource management initiative. British Journal of Health Care Computing 8(5): 6

Benner P 1984 From novice to expert: excellence and power in clinical nursing practice. Addison Wesley, Menlo Park

Benner P, Wrubel J 1989 The primacy of caring. Addison Wesley, Menlo Park

Brown P, Warren L 1991 Implementing clinical audit. The British Journal of Health Care Computing 8(5): 14–18

Bryson D M 1991 The computer literate nurse. Computers in Nursing 9(3): 100–107

Chandler D 1990 The educational ideology of the computer. British Journal of Educational Technology 21(3): 165–174

Evans D, Evans M, Greaves D 1991 Adding life to years: problems in planning for health gain. International Journal of Health Care Quality Assurance 4(1): 13–20

Ford J 1990 Computers and nursing: possibilities for transforming nursing. Computers in Nursing 8(4): 160–164

Graves J R, Corcoran S 1989 The study of nursing informatics. Image: Journal of Nursing Scholarship 21(4): 227–231

Jones B T 1991 Building nursing expert systems using automated rule induction. Computers in Nursing 9(2): 52–60

Jones B T, Buchanan M 1989 Relieving the bottlenecks in ward activity monitoring through IT. Information Technology in Nursing 1(2): 27–31

MacIntyre A 1985 After virtue: a study in moral theory, 2nd edn. Duckworth, London

Noddings N 1986 Caring: a feminine approach to ethics and moral education. University of California Press, Berkeley

Plant J A 1983 Is nursing confidential? In: Scholes M, Bryant Y, Barber B (eds) The impact of computers on nursing: an international review. Proceedings of the IFIP-IMIA workshop on the impact of computers on nursing 1982. North-Holland, Amsterdam

Redmond D T 1983 An overview of the development of National Health Service computing. In: Scholes M, Bryant Y, Barber B (eds) The impact of computers on nursing. North-Holland, Amsterdam

Reverby S M 1987 Ordered to care—the dilemma of American nursing 1850–1945. Cambridge University Press, Cambridge

Sinclair V G 1990 Potential effects of decision support systems on the role of the nurse. Computers in Nursing 8(2): 60–65

Squire P 1983 The nurse manager and the computer. In: Scholes M, Bryant Y, Barber B (eds) The impact of computers on nursing. North Holland, Amsterdam

Strength D E, Keen-Payne R 1991 Computerised patient care documentation: educational applications in the baccalaureate curriculum. Computers in Nursing 9(1): 22–26

Taylor R, Cameron C 1990 Resource Management systems for nursing managers. Information Technology in Nursing 1(4): 65–67

Walsh M, Cortez F 1991 Quality assurance system must balance functionality with data security. Computers in Nursing 9(1): 27–28

Warren L 1991 Seminar report: primary care. Report from PHCSG Conference. The British Journal of Health Care computing 8(5): 10

Watson J 1985 Nursing: the philosophy and science of caring. Colorado Associated University Press, Boulder

Index

Action
  aesthetic–expressive reality domain, 23, 24, 25
  cognitive–instrumental reality domain, 23, 24, 25
  as communication, 23–26
Added life, 187–188
American Psychiatric Association, DSM-III-R, 11
Anxiety, and computer use, 146, 147
Artificial intelligence (AI), 3
Attitude formation, to information technology, 146, 171
Attributes
  attribute values distinction, 47–48
  descriptor set establishment, critical incident technique, 48
  free listing, 48–49
  known, unknown factor assumption, 63
  listing frequency and importance, 48–49
  value elicitation, 49–50
  patient-focused interviews, 50
Audits
  patient care, 107–108
  patient types, 109–110
Authenticity, action, and aesthetic–expressive domain, 24
Automated rule induction, 65

Bevan, Aneurin, and NHS, 73
Biopsies, computer analysis, 3
Budget monitoring, 79

CANIS system, 102
Care
  and caring, 177
  improvement, and nursing informatics, 178–179
  see also Health care; Patient care
Caring, 177
  different patients/different responses, 189
  Nodding's views, 188–189
City life
  instability and unpredictability, 20
  space/mores, 17, 18
Classification, and nursing knowledge, 12
Clinical reasoning
  abductive inference, 60–61
  hypothetical–deductive model, 56, 59
Cognition
  and fact assumption, 61–62
  heuristic, 57, 66
  higher
    deliberate, 58
    use by nurses, 57–62
  of nurses
    and attributes, 56
    understanding of, 55–57
Cognitive model, reliability measures, 55
Common nursing language, 29–31, 42, 50
  demonstration exercise, 30
Communication
  and action, 23–26
  and information technology, 152
Community Health Information Classification and Coding (CHIC) project, 83–84
Community Information Systems Project (NHS, 1991), 83, 85

Community Information Systems
    Project (NHS, 1991) *(contd)*
  data collection principles, 85
Computer literacy
  domains, Minnesota Educational
    Consortium, 181–182
  nurses, 99
  teaching, ethical concepts, 181–182
Computer-assisted learning (CAL),
    143, 145, 154
  package evaluation, 148
  student confidence in use, 165, 167
Computerphobia, 171
Computers
  access to, 168
  advantages/disadvantages, patient
    care, 186–187
  anxiety and use, 146, 147
  classification of users, 157
  culture dangers, 185, 189
  experience/use, student nurses,
    166–168
  hands-on experience, 155
  and human origin of information
    (Chandler), 184–185
  low use, by students, 168
  in nursing, 129–137
    benefits, 136
    clinical applications, 131
    competencies approach, 132–133
    content approach, 131–132
    future nursing practice, 133–134
    nursing science approach, 133–135
    practitioner preparation, 135–137
    use difficulties, 136–137
    user competencies, 132
    user resistance, 137
  personal use, 167
  school use, 167, 168
  student knowledge of availability,
    168
Conceptual schema hypothesis,
    patient assessment, 64, 66
Condition–action pairs, expert
    systems, 119
Confidentiality
  information technology, 154
  and nursing, 180–181
Cues
  importance in patient assessment,
    56–57
  in nurse's working memory, 60, 64
Current Medical Information and
    Terminology (CMIT), 12

Curricula, nursing
  development, and IT, 147–148,
    150–152
  information technology, 139–157

Data
  and information, context dependent
    distinctions, 88–89
  selection and use bias, 94–95
Data Protection Act (1984), 98, 154
Decision making
  choice phase, 90–91
  critical thinking/analysis, 153
  descriptive model (Simon), 89–90
  and information, 74–77
  and information technology, 99
  Kepner & Tregoe, 92–93
  matrix, 93
  nurse's influence, 142
  patient assessment, 63–64, 65–66
  process, 65–66
  rational, 88–93
    nursing process, 91–92
    prescriptive model, 91–92
    stages, 91
    use problems, 92
  stages, 89
  structured/unstructured, 91
  team, 90, 92
  and theories of choice, 74–75, 76
  Thomas model, 92
Design, and decision making, 90
Diagnosis
  and expert systems, 126
  and low-level attributes, 9
  nursing, 186
    structure, 59
  psychological studies, 61
Diagnostic and Statistical Manual for
    Mental Disorders (DSM-III-R),
    11
Discriminant function analysis, 65
Disease
  illness distinction, 9
  nominalist approach, 8
  and patient attributes, 8
Duty, and nursing, 35

ECGs, computer analysis, 2
Education
  critical thinking/analysis, 153
  and information technology, 143–144
    post-registration, 174
    Welsh study implications, 173–174

Education *(contd)*
  nursing and IT combination
    problems, 147, 150–152
  traditional
    information technology imped-
      ence, 143
    ward-based information systems,
      167
EEGs, computer analysis, 2
Efficiency
  action, and cognitive–instrumental
    domain, 24
  in nursing, historical aspects,
    183–184
Employee control, and informatics, 22
Estrangement, and society trans-
    formation, 18
Ethics
  and informatics, 179–183
  and information technology, 153–154
Expert nurses, 46
  cognition, and proficient nurses'
    cognition, 63, 64
Expert systems, 43, 186
  condition–action pairs, 119
  cost-effectiveness, 125
  and diagnostic skills, 125
  as learning aids, 116
  nursing practice, 141
  prototyping cycle, 120–121
    construction stage, 120
    definition stage, 120
    testing stage, 120–121
  software
    development, 119–121
    selection, 118–119
Expertise
  and competency, 46
  experiential element, 186
  intuitive, 186
  and problem solving systems,
    185–186
Experts
  and informatics, 20, 23
  and knowledge, 45–47

Formalisation, and co-operation, 22

General practitioners, patient data
    confidentiality, 181
Griffiths Report, 73–74, 159
GUIDON, 61

Health care
  automated systems, 129–130
  coded language (NHS), 84
  costs, 73
  and health gain, 187–189
  monitoring, 79–80
Health gain
  groups and individuals, 187
  and patient outcomes, 187–188
  and technology, 187–189
Health problems
  classification/nomenclature, 10–12
  nursing approach, 9–10
HELP (Health Evaluation through
    Logic Processing), 3, 4
Hospital information support sytems,
    169, 170
Hospital statistics, and Florence
    Nightingale, 57, 71–72
Hypotheses
  diagnostic, 60
  testing, 58, 60

Illness, disease distinction, 9
Impartiality, in nursing, 35
Inference
  abductive (Pople), in clinical
    reasoning, 60–61
  backward-chaining process, 119
  logical/deductive, and nursing
    expertise, 58
Informatics
  code of conduct (Squires), 182–183
  and employee control, 22
  ethics, 179–183
  heterogeneous strengths, 19–20
  normative view, 23, 25
  and nursing curricula, 152–153
  and optimistic attitude, 19, 20, 23
  perspectives, 21
  and romantic attitude, 18–19, 20, 23
  term origin, 1
  see also Data; Information; Infor-
    mation technology; Medical
    informatics; Nursing
    informatics
Information
  collection and use, 76–81
  in community setting, 81
  cost and value, 88
  and decision making, 74–77
    model, 75
  excess/useless, 76–77
  humans as processors, 94
  interpretation

196 INDEX

Information *(contd)*
  and action, 104–105
  message or dialogue, 104, 105
  managerial requirements, 80
  nature and role, 88–89
  need for, 159
  nursing requirements, 78
  operational requirements, 80, 81–82
    definition, 82
    and off-the-shelf systems, 82
  organisational flow, 78, 79, 81
  organisation's requirements
    analysis, 93–95
    determination methodology, 95–97
    social/behavioural aspects, 96–97
    software, 96
    structure/process/documentation, 96
  other organisations, 81
  person-centred systems, 82–85
  prioritisation, 80
  processing, contingent/goal-directed, 62
  requirements
    analysis/evaluation, 71–99
    organisation of, 80–81
  service objectives, 78–80
  strategic requirements, 81
  strategy, development, 77–78
  use levels, 80–81
  volume, and nursing, 58
Information technology
  anxiety, 146, 147
  and communication, 152
  confidentiality, 154
  courses
    evaluation, 156
    monitoring/evaluation, 148
    planning, 146–147
    teaching, 150–151
  curriculum
    content, 149–154
    development, 147–148
  and education, 143–144
  and ethics, 153–154
  formal educational opportunities, 169–170
  and management, 141–142
  neutrality, 184–187
  nurse role preparation, 160–162
  in nursing curricula, 139–157
    integration, 150–152
    need for, 140–144
  nursing involvement, 160–161
  and nursing practice, 141
  and nursing science, 140–141
  organisation and teaching, Welsh study, 171
  participants, 144–146
  perceived relevance, 146, 151–152
  and research, 142–143
  sharing, 156
  skills levels, 148
  student attitudes, Welsh study, 171
  student nurse's use, 159–175
  students, 145–146
    attitude formation, 146
    skills assessment, 155–156
  teachers, 144–146
  teaching methods, 154–155
  terminology, student understanding, 169, 170
  see also Informatics; Information
Information technology system
  benefits analysis, 98–99
  evaluation, 98–99
  features, 97–98
  hardware, 97–98
  see also Expert systems; Nursing information systems (NISs)
Intelligence, and decision-making, 89–90
Interference phenomenom, life-world/system, and nursing informatics, 25–26
International Classification of Diseases (ICD), 11
Intuition, and nursing expertise, 58

Jargon, and shared understanding, 42
Justice, action, moral–practical reality domain, 24

Knowledge
  codified, 39
  cognitive, 44–45
  deep, 44
  descriptive, 44
    microlevel, 49–50
  holder identification, 45–47
  inter-expert inconsistencies, 46
  practical dimensions, 39, 46–47
  practitioner, 44–45
  processing, 44–45
  professional, 38
  semi-codified process (Eraut), 39
  surface, 44
  technical, 39

Knowledge *(contd)*
 theoretical dimensions, 46–47
 top-level, elicitation, 47–48
 types, 38–40
 see also Nursing knowledge;
   Processing knowledge
Korner Report (1984), 89, 159

Language, nursing, uniform, 29–31, 42, 50
Learning
 and being taught, 38
 by experience, 36–38
 computer-assisted (CAL), 143, 145, 148, 154, 165, 167
 ethical aspects, 37–38
 organisational, 112–113
Life-world/system, reconciliation, 26

Management
 information systems (MIS), 90–91
 and information technology, 80, 141–142
 scientific (Taylorism), 22
Maslow's hierarchy of needs, 7
Medical descriptions, hierarchical levels, 8–9
Medical informatics, 2–7
 data applications, 2–3
 definitions, 4–7
  Braude, 4
  Greenes & Shortliffe, 4
  Möhr, 4
  Reichertz, 4
  Van Bemmel, 5–6, 13
 historical aspects, 2–4
 and humanistic approach to medicine, 6
 information applications, 2, 3
 knowledge applications, 2, 3
 nursing informatics relationship, 14–15
 objects of study, 6
 phase merging, 3–4
 working model (Van Bemmel), 5–6
Medicine, humanistic approach, and medical informatics, 6
Memory, working, and nursing, 60, 64
MeSH (Medical Subject Headings), 12
Minimum data sets (MDS), 50, 153, 160
 construction, 42
 nursing, 13–14, 134–135
Minnesota Educational Consortium, computer literacy domains, 181–182

MYCIN, 61

National Library of Medicine (US), Unified Medical Language System, 12
National Vocational Qualifications, 35
Needs hierarchy (Maslow), 7
NHS
 Aneurin Bevan's views, 73
 Centre for Coding and Classification, 84
 Community Information Systems Project (1991), 83, 85
 and demographic changes, 73
 resource management, 160, 169, 170
Nightingale, Florence, 57, 71–72
 on confidentiality, 180
Norton scales, pressure sore risk assessment, 117
Nurses
 computer knowledge need, 170, 171
 computer literacy, 99
 patient relationships, 178
Nursing
 core concern/activities, 10
 definition difficulty, 31
 and disease low-level attributes, 10
 duty and impartiality, 35
 function of, 32–35
 health problem approach, 9–10
 image/identity, 25
 information requirements, 78
 knowledge-based (expert) systems, 14
 legal accountability, 33
 moral nature, 177–178
 observable/unobservable skills, 36
 and patient trust, 34
 performance criteria, 32–33
 phenomenon, 30, 31–35
 professional, conceptualisation/analytical skills, 36
 purpose of, 35–36
 self-regulation, 33
Nursing diagnosis *see* Diagnosis
Nursing informatics
 benefits, 178–179
 and care improvement, 178–179
 and confidentiality, 180–181
 definition, 180
 definitions, 72–73
 founding principles, 7–15
 goals, 72
 growth, 75–76

Nursing Information Management
   (Graves & Corcoran), 25
Nursing information systems (NISs)
   benefits, 110
   clinical practice support, 101–114
   computer-assisted, 103–104
   development, 106–107
   engineering, 13
   existing practice automation, 105
   formal and informal, 103–104
   and informatics, 13
   new structures and methodologies,
      prototyping, 113
   nurse interfaces, 13
   nursing system in use, 102–105
   requirements, 97, 102
Nursing knowledge
   formalisation, 29–40
      definition/limits, 41–42
      key issues, 43
      methodological issues, 47–66
      rationale, 42–43
      nature, 30–31
      see also Knowledge; Practitioner
         knowledge
Nursing language see Common
   nursing language
Nursing phenomena, data, 134–135
Nursing practice
   analysis, and IT systems, 98
   and computers, 129–137
   costing, 184
   in future, 133–134
      preparation for, 135–137
   humanistic approach, 19–20
   and information technology, 141
   and nursing information systems,
      101–114
   and problem solving systems,
      185–186
   technical innovations, 134
Nursing process
   computer-assisted care planning
      systems, 108–109
   data collection/use, ethical aspects,
      181
   rationale decision making, 91–92
Nursing records, purpose, 84–85
Nursing science see Science of nursing

Opportunity seeking, and decision
   making, 89–90
Organisations
   activity outcomes, review, 112–113

   information requirements, 93–97
Output/activity monitoring, 79–80

Patient care
   computer advantages/
      disadvantages, 186–187
   goals evaluation, 109–110
   plan structure, 108–109
   planning
      and audit, 107–108
      expert systems, 126
      model, 110–111
      questions facing nurses, 106, 107
      standards, 111–112
      monitoring, 109–110
Patients
   assessment, decision making point,
      63–64
   classification, 184
      prototype approach, 58–59, 60
   computed health history, 84
   data confidentiality, 180–183
   nurse relationships, 34, 178
   outcome measurements, 188
   simulated assessment, computer-
      assisted, 53–55
   trust in nurses, 34
PAWMEX, 116–126
   completed knowledge base, 121
   components, 121
   help facility, 121, 122, 123
   independent evaluation, 123–124
   inter-user reliability, 123
   nursing implications, 124–125
   references/bibliography, 123
   response screen, 121, 122
   software development, 119–121
   system operation, 121–123
Perception
   absolute, 21
   analysis (Merleau-Ponty), 21
   and knowledge building, 21
Personal development,
   self-evaluation, 154
Philosophy, and informatics, 17–26
Pneumonia, attributes, 9
Practitioner knowledge, 44–45
Pressure sores
   extrinsic aetiological factors, 116
   intrinsic aetiological factors, 117
   management, 117–118
   NHS costs, 124
   research problem, 118
   risk assessment

Pressure sores *(contd)*
  PAWMEX, 116–126
  and problem solving skills, 117
  software development, 119–121
  software selection, 118–119
Problem identification, and decision making, 89–90
Problem solving
  behaviour, human, 95
  group exercises, 155
  pressure risk assessment, 117
  rational, 92–93
  systems, professional practice/expertise effects, 185–186
Problem space, problem solving, 95
Process tracing
  cognition studies, 52
  simulated patient assessment, computer-assisted, 53–55
Processing knowledge
  analysing and modelling, 55–57
  contingent/goal-directed, 62
  formalisation, 51–52
Professional characteristics, identification by function, 33–35
Project 2000 (UKCC, 1986), 115–116
Protocol analysis, verbal, 51–52
Psychiatry/clinical medicine, attribute and nominal views, comparisons, 8–9

Quality, of service, monitoring, 80
Quality assurance, 141–142
  and patient data confidentiality, 180
Quality improvement, continuous, 142

Rationalism, and agreement on informatics, 23
Read Clinical Classification Scheme, 50
Research, and information technology, 142–143
Resource management
  and care improvement, 179
  historical aspects, 183–184
  initiatives, 104, 169, 170
  NHS, 160
  and nursing managers, 183–184
Risk assessment
  by nurses, 54–55
  experienced nurses, 55
  see also Pressure sores

Schizophrenia, description, 8–9

Schools of nursing, IT policies, (Welsh study), 168, 169
Science of nursing
  and computers, 133–135
  and information technology, 140–141
Self-evaluation, personal development, 154
Service objectives
  information, 78–80
  monitoring provision, 79–80
Smears, computer analysis, 3
SNOMED (Systemised Nomenclature for Medicine), 12
Society
  as city, 17–18, 23
  as village, 18, 23
Society metaphor, and informatics, 17–19
Solutions, evaluation, and decision making, 90
Strategy for Nursing (DoH, 1989), 162
Student assessment, information technology skills, 155–156
Student nurses, computer system requirement definition, 165
Student nurses, and information technology, 159–175
  Welsh study *see* Welsh study
  see also Curricula, nursing; Education; Information technology

Task environment, problem solving, 95
Taylorism (scientific management), 22
TDS system, and medical/nursing care, 3, 7
Teachers, informatics knowledge and study, 130–131
Technology
  achievements, negativism/indifference, 19, 23
  health care/health gain, 187–189
Thinking
  critical, and nurse education, 153
  shaping, and technology, 185

UK, Resource Management Initiative (RMI), 30–31, 104
Unified Medical Language System (UMLS), 12, 50

Verbal protocol analysis, 51–52
  reliability/validity, 52

Video, interactive, in education, 143, 154
Village life
   operating laws and regularities, 20
   space/mores, 18

Waterlow scale, pressure sore risk assessment, 117
Welsh study, 162–174
   computer experience/use, 166–168
   data collection, 163–164
   IT organisation and teaching, 171
   methods, 163
   nurse education implications, 173–174
   objectives, 163
   recommendations, 174–175
   results, 164–174
   and student ages, 164
   students' knowledge of IT, 164–165
   sample, 163, 164
   student nurse IT exposure, 164
   students' attitudes to IT, 171
   students' expressed needs, 172
WHO, International Classification of Diseases, 11
WiseOne
   expert system shell, 118–119
   modules, 119
Word processing, 167
Working memory, nurses, 60, 64
Working for Patients (1989), 74, 89, 160
Wound management
   PAWMEX, 116–126
   software development, 119–121
   software selection, 118–119